PLAYING WITHOUT A PARTNER

PLAYING WITHOUT A PARTNER

A SINGLES GUIDE TO SEX, DATING, AND HAPPINESS

MEGAN STUBBS, EdD

CLEiS
PRESS

Published in the United States by Cleis Press, an imprint of Start Mid-night, LLC, 221 River Street, Ninth Floor, Hoboken, New Jersey 07030.

Printed in the United States
Cover design: Jennifer Do
Cover image: Shutterstock
Text design: Frank Wiedemann

First Edition.
10 9 8 7 6 5 4 3 2 1

Trade paper ISBN: 978-1-62778-304-0
E-book ISBN: 978-1-62778-517-4

TABLE OF CONTENTS

To You, the reader.

Thank you

WHO ARE YOU?

While many of us heard nursery rhymes about the butcher, the baker, and the candlestick maker, we never heard about the sexologist. Perhaps it was too hard to rhyme with? Either way, it's a real job.

My story began in middle school. I was always that friend you could go to for your sexual or relationship concerns. Inappropriate? Pervert? Slut? Maybe for some, but either way, I was motivated. Mind you, all of us were learning and discovering new things for ourselves, but I was always the one reading up on what was going on "down there." I remember going to the bookstore with my mom and sneakily walking into the "relationship" section of the store, *only* when no one else was in the aisle, as if I'd be caught there. As soon as someone walked by, I quickly did a 180 and pretended to peruse the exercise and fitness books. Lucky save on the store layout!

I credit my mom with my invaluable and early love of reading. I recall many memories of sitting on her lap listening to her read to me, instilling a love for the knowledge that books imparted. Of course, those books mostly led me to believe that animals talked and much of life would end happily ever after. Nonetheless, I became a bibliophile. I developed the ability to not only read quickly, but retain the information I had just read.

Fast-forward to high school. I always had a knack for science, mainly biology. Incidentally, the only AP exam I passed was AP Biology. For those who may not know, AP courses are set at an advanced pace and allow you to potentially earn college credit while still in high school, if you pass their comprehensive exam. When it came time to apply for college, I chose Grand Valley State University. It was close to home, had a great reputation for the sciences, and gave me college credit for my passed AP exam. I was in.

Lofty dreams had me set on the pre-med path, but unbeknownst to me, chemistry would be my downfall—or actually the catalyst to make me search for something more. I sucked at chemistry. It was embarrassing. It was the reason that I knew I wasn't going to be able to pursue a medical degree. Cue depression and dashed dreams. Where was I to head? What was I going to do with a biology degree? Where could I use my knowledge of how life works, evolution, and behavior? It only took one trip to the grocery store to make me realize where my true talents lay: sex.

Next time you're in the grocery store, casually look at what all of the glossy magazines that are strategically placed in the stands are telling you. Almost every magazine has something pertaining to sex. Whether it's five secrets to help you blow your man's mind, or ten new ways to feel better about your appearance, it is all about sex.

I graduated with my bachelor's in biology and immediately started my studies to become a sexologist. I went to one of the few graduate schools in the country that grants advanced degrees in the study of human sexuality, and I've never looked back.

So before we delve any deeper into the tale of my career path, let me define for you what exactly the terms *sexology* and *sexologist* mean.

Sexology is the study of human sexuality. So, not surprisingly, a sexologist is someone who has received an extensive education and training in the field of human sexuality. And as it is an ever-changing and growing field, they are someone who is continually accessing the latest research in human sexuality to better their own understanding and to strive to provide the most accurate and up-to-date information.

Sex school was nothing like I could have ever imagined. I never counted on the breadth of the education I would receive there. I was exposed to things I had never heard of, let alone seen! But it was all part of the education. Exposing myself to these different aspects of sexuality made me realize that there truly is no "normal" ANYTHING. Sexuality is subjective. Our culture, family upbringing, and religious convictions all go into shaping who we are and how we think, as well as how we feel about sex. This education through exposure helped me find out what my buttons—sexual hang-ups—were and how to come to terms with them. No one is going to like everything, and I'm not saying I do either, but I have learned to be impartial and open to everyone else's unique perspective on sex and sexuality, because who am I to judge?

One of the most common questions I was asked when I first started attending school was "Umm . . . so do you, like, have sex homework?" And the short answer was, "Yeah, it's sex school!" Like any other university we had books, videos, guest speakers, and field trips, but that wasn't why people were asking me. They wanted to know if we had actual sex in class.

Well, in order to be well versed in anything, you have to practice it. Would a chef be able to cook without having learned how to cut vegetables and operate in the kitchen? Same notion applies here. I experienced my own sexual journey, which is by no means over yet, but which opened me up to many of the possibilities of what sex can be. And I'm not just speaking about PV (penis in vagina) sex. A common phrase I say to people is "Put on your own oxygen mask before assisting others." (I come by it honestly, having a mom who is a flight attendant.) If I'm not comfortable and secure in my own sexuality, how on earth am I supposed to help someone else with theirs? So did we bang in class? Much of our homework was research in the form of "me-search" and self-driven at home, outside of class. Very few exercises were partnered ones, sorry to disappoint. No class orgies were had.

Fast forward to present time, and I have spent the last decade educating and normalizing the conversation around sex.

Life can take you to many places you never thought you'd visit. For me, 2017 was a particularly interesting year. I had just broken up with my latest partner, and I decided to enact what I called "Man Ban 2017." This was when I would reset and revitalize my life without the influence of men. I became the sexless sexologist. While this was a decision I essentially made overnight, it wasn't as if my life hadn't been building to that point. I had become accustomed to how my dating cycles would repeat themselves, and they weren't bringing me any closer to my goals.

Tough lessons in my twenties showed me that I had to be more protective of what I put out into the dating environment. Many men who found out what I did had some kind of negative reaction. Whether it was objectification, exploitation, or using me as a conquest, it was never anything good. This went far beyond the nervousness of the "bringing you home to meet the family" conversation. I knew that if I couldn't find a partner who was not only cool with what I did, but truly supportive, I wasn't going to have lasting happiness. So the ban came into place.

It wasn't as if I was missing out by not having partnered sex. I did miss out on those connections that are only found when you are with another person, of course, but they weren't strong enough to sway me from my course. I was already my own best lover, so it wasn't hard to find sexual satisfaction with myself. And I had plenty of past experiences to draw from. I'd had my fair share of Mr. Right Nows.

That year I saw great leaps of progress in my personal and professional life. I was free from the time and effort it takes to cultivate a relationship with another. All of the time I had now was spent on bettering myself. And time spent on yourself is never time wasted. The clearer my intentions became, the more I was able to map out a plan to make my goals become a reality. I revisited old hobbies and thrived in the success I had with them. I formulated what my ideal relationship would look like and focused on the details so that I would be better able to recognize it when they crossed my path. I connected with friends and lived my best life.

I'm a little older now, but the work put in during that time is still with me today.

You've hit the trifecta: I'm a sexologist, I'm single, and

I'm so excited to impart everything that I've learned over the years of on-the-job education and off-the-clock research. After the many false starts and stories that friends proclaimed, "would be a good chapter in a book," I'm excited for you to learn how to lean on yourself when you are reserving a table for one.

WHO IS THIS BOOK FOR?

Inclusivity

This book is written from my perspective, which is that of a heterosexual cisgender woman. But most of this information can be applied to anyone of any gender or sexual orientation. This is also true of someone just beginning their sexual journey or a frequent flier. I've tried to incorporate accessible, actionable components that can be applied to your life as soon as you read them. It's not all encompassing. That would be a much larger book! But I've tried to assemble some of the key aspects, in my opinion, of what is important for a single person to keep front of mind in order to live their best life.

And with that being said, feel free to jump around. While this book can be read front to back, you are more than welcome to visit an area of interest outside of the chronological order. I hope you'd use this as your guide to empowerment and sexual satisfaction, and as a blueprint for building a life that you're happy to lead, single or otherwise.

As you can imagine, when you have a sexologist writing a book, you're bound to have some terms that may not be familiar to you. There may also be some terms that you've heard in passing, so I just wanted to lay a few of them out here.

Partner: This word can be used in a variety of ways. This

could refer to someone that was a one-time sex partner. This could refer to someone you have a new relationship with, or it could mean someone that you're thinking about having a romantic encounter with. This isn't always indicative of someone that you have a long-term relationship with.

Play: Did you smile when you read the title? Sometimes when you want to have covert conversations about sexual activity, you can substitute the word *play*. For instance, at brunch you can talk about your date the previous night and rate whether or not the play was satisfactory. Perfectly proper sounding conversation.

As a last note on language: I have sometimes used terms like *men* and *women* when referring to types of bodies or sex, but I would be remiss if I didn't include trans men and women, nonbinary folks, and intersex folks. Where applicable, I've tried to use terminology reflective of specific parts rather than blanket gender statements. Speaking from a heteronormative place does a disservice to the wide range of people in existence, and I want to make sure as many people as possible are seen and given advice within these pages.

Single Audience

This book was written with the assumption that you are not already in a committed relationship. I think so often when it comes to books on sex, relationships, and how to improve them, there is the underlying assumption that you're already with a longer-term partner! The strategies recommended often rely on you having the preexisting safety of good, open communication in that relationship, or a certain level of intimacy and trust with your partner. But single people, whose partners may either be brand new or nonexistent, don't necessarily have that luxury. It's just you and me here!

Since I'm assuming that you're single, you're going to be your own partner! I hope that through exploring this book you will gain greater insight on what it means to be single. I want to empower you to take charge of your life, both as a single person and a future partnered one, so that you're equipped to handle anything that life throws at you. The growth you do here will benefit you in the years to come. I've said it before, but it's worth repeating: I wholly believe that time spend on yourself is never time wasted.

The confident single person is already living and building the life they want. They aren't seeking to fill holes, no pun intended. You don't need someone else to complete you, you are already a whole person. If this isn't you yet, we will hopefully get you there soon.

Always keep this in mind: Adding a healthy relationship to an already fulfilled life should be the metaphorical cherry on top. Of course there will be days when hearing your friend say the word *husband/partner* will cause your eye to twitch and tears to fall, but remember all of the possibility and opportunity you are poised for.

Whether singlehood is a temporary or permanent status, create the life you want, surround yourself with things and people that bring you love and joy, and be grateful for what you have at this time and in this place.

JOURNALING

As you go through this book, consider keeping a journal as a companion, there to help you document your journey as you discover new things about yourself or feel compelled to jot your ideas down. I'm a huge fan of bullet journals. They help keep my life and my sanity on track. Despite being nearly glued to electronic devices, there is something about paper and pen that I love. I often have to tell myself that I don't need more pens, even if there's a sale on the very cute twenty-four-pack of dual-ended pens that I'm looking at in a separate window. (I don't have any brush tips yet. Bitch, you don't need them!)

Maybe you're not like me and digital is life for you. That's okay too! Don't get caught up in the medium. Maybe you're a cocktail napkin, back of receipt, Post-it Note kind of person. That's perfectly okay! The important thing is that you start the process of getting your thoughts down. Research suggests[1] that people who have a journaling practice are happier in life and have less stress.

SAY IT LOUD, SAY IT PROUD

I'm single. That simple phase can be said with all of the confidence in the world or with shame, like someone who feels like they're wearing a gigantic scarlet *S* on their forehead.

Whether you're newly single or have been living the life for a while, there can be strong emotions associated with this relationship status. As with anything, you will have good days and bad days, but singlehood should not be treated like a prison sentence. Take time to reflect on your situation and realize that you have so much, if not more, opportunity and

1 Joshua M. Smyth et al. "Online Positive Affect Journaling in the Improvement of Mental Distress and Well-Being in General Medical Patients With Elevated Anxiety Symptoms: A Preliminary Randomized Controlled Trial," *JMIR Mental Health*, 5, no. 4 (October 12, 2018), https://doi.org/10.2196/11290.

freedom than your paired or married friends. Together we will reveal aspects of the life you may be overlooking and see what new practices you can incorporate into your life.

Yes, you are alone in the sense that you are not romantically involved with anyone right now, but that doesn't mean it's time to wallow in self-pity and binge eat Häagen-Dazs by the pint. Being single is as much of a choice as being in a relationship or being married. So the next time a family member says, "When are you going to get married?" tell them that you're busy living your life to the fullest. The single and confident person isn't looking to settle with just anyone—they have high standards. They don't associate their relationship status with their worth. Your life as a single person is perfect for embarking on a new journey or opportunity. Think of the freedom you enjoy without having to consider someone else's schedule. Adventure could be around the next corner.

STATS ON BEING SINGLE

The 2017 US Census Bureau's American community survey reported that more than 110 million US residents—almost 45% of adults aged eighteen or older—were divorced, widowed, or had never been married.[2] That's almost half the marriage-aged population! But when you constantly find yourself as one of the only few single people amongst your friend group, it can seem like that number is wrong.

If I can be frankly honest with you: If you had asked me in my early twenties what my life would look like in ten years, I

---

2 Bella DePaulo, "There's Never Been a Better Time to be Single," CNN Health, last modified March 9, 2018, https://www.cnn.com/2018/01/05/health/single-people-partner/index.html.

would have absolutely said that I would have been partnered, if not married, by now. Traversing these years single, while all of your peer group has seemingly left you behind, can be incredibly discouraging. When your activities with your friend group have shifted from all nighters and parties to daylight activities and second birthday parties, it can feel like a jolt. Where did the time go, and what happened to me? If this is speaking to you, I have to let you in on something else, too.

While there is nothing wrong about feeling this way, I want to draw your attention to the tone of these thoughts. We are products of our mind. What we think becomes our reality. Extrapolating from that, if we view this time of singledom in a lamentable way, this will subconsciously permeate our day-to-day life. More basically put, if you're sad about being single, this will undermine your well-being.

I'm speaking of prolonged sadness. This is of course separate from mourning the loss of someone or the end of a relationship. Grief is natural and part of life. What I'm talking about is the everyday wake up mood of, *ugh, here I am, still single.*

According to a study done on Match.com, "75% of Gen Z and 69% of Millennials believe they will find the kind of love they want."[3] So this should be heartening. You aren't alone in the hopes to one day find a partnership that is right for you.

In the meantime, we want to shift, jumpstart, refresh, and revive our life perspective, so we can see the good that is already around us and the good that is just around the corner, waiting to be discovered.

---

3 "Singles In America," Match.com, last modified July 30, 2019, https://match.mediaroom.com/2019-07-30-Singles-in-America-Match-Releases-Ninth-Annual-Study-on-U-S-Single-Population.

WHAT SOCIETY SAYS ABOUT BEING SINGLE

The reaction society has to single people is often one of "Oh poor you." Society imagines the office spinster at the company holiday party. It makes singles the subject of discussions about hooking up said single people so they don't have to be alone anymore.

Even at family gatherings this can happen—or maybe *especially* at family gatherings. For me, it's my grandma constantly asking me if I have a man in my life. "You know, a lot of men would be happy with a woman like you," Grandma counsels. Yea, I know Grandma! I'm a catch! But what kind of man would make me happy? I haven't come across him yet, so here we are. This is commonly followed by the discussion of having children, which Grandma still doesn't believe is out of the cards for me. Only fur babies here, Grandma!

But, while society may have these perceptions about the single population, when we actually look at the numbers, many people report to be content. One study published in *The Journals of Gerontology* found that as people aged, their "satisfaction with being single increased," and likewise they found that younger generations also tended to be more satisfied with a single relationship status.[4] Unfortunately, even with many finding peace with their solo traverse in life, still the stigma around singlehood continues.

Oh the pressure to be partnered! For many people in the

---

4 Anne Boger and Oliver Huxhold, "The Changing Relationship between Partnership Status and Loneliness: Effects Related to Aging and Historical Time," *The Journals of Gerontology: Series B* 75, no. 7 (December 22, 2018): 1423–1432, https://doi.org/https://doi.org/10.1093/geronb/gby153.

past, finding a relationship was the way to gain their independence, in a way. It was the norm to have women stay at home until they could finally go out on their own to explore the world—under the watchful eye of their partners. To be married was to have an exalted position in society. Fortunately, these days we can be regarded as adults without having to say "I do," but expectations haven't fully shifted from those traditional values, which are so ingrained into our being.

And marriage still affords certain privileges to couples, both legally and monetarily, that single folks don't receive. Not to mention some married couples' second incomes, or access to a spouse's health insurance plan. Society is set up to benefit the partnered. Only married people have access to seeing their partner if they're in a hospital and unresponsive. Testifying against your spouse is protected. Even those window salespeople will only make a pitch if both you AND your spouse are present. "Will Mr. Stubbs be joining us?" Absolutely not.

In some cultures, to be single is to be looked upon with disgrace. What's wrong with you? Why doesn't anyone want to be with you? Such thinking can leave singles feeling less about themselves. When the status of coupledom is more important than the individual, the individual can become invisible. And for women: when your culture expects you to be a wife and a mother, it's considered weird when you're not.

Singles can also be made to feel "less than" in smaller, less blatant ways. Who is the first person relegated to sleeping on the couch during family gatherings? Spoiler (or not really): It's the single person! Just because you don't "need" the space for you and your partner. Or, maybe your partnered friends shift to having lunch with you since they prefer to dine with other couples at night, rather than having a threesome dinner date. Perhaps you're expected to pay twice as much when friends "split" costs by couple. Maybe it's just having to check the "single" box every time you do your taxes.

A study looking at cultural bias against singles in *Current Directions of Psychological Science*[5] researched the perceptions one thousand people had when it came to married and single people. Unsurprisingly, sentiments like happy, loyal, mature, and loving were said when it came to married individuals. But when it came to the perceptions of single people, the praise fell short. Sentiments like immature, self-centered, insecure, lonely, and unhappy were perceived by the respondents.

But value shouldn't be reliant on who you're with. Rather, it should be reliant on who you are.

The perception is that single people are sad, lonely creatures longing for the day to finally have a partner so they can matter to the world. Is that the reality though? Of course not! Many singles report having fulfilling lives, cultivating a life that brings them joy. You can want to be in a relationship as a single person and ALSO have a happy life as a single person. Those two ideas are not mutually exclusive.

If we use the assumption that single people are all of those negative traits we listed above, we must live with a lot of grumpy people. According to the US Census Bureau, there have never been more single people in this country than now!

---

5 Bella M. DePaulo and Wendy L. Morris, "The Unrecognized Stereotyping and Discrimination Against Singles," *Current Directions in Psychological Science* 13, no. 5 (October 2006): 251–254, https://doi.org/https://doi.org/10.1111%2Fj.1467-8721.2006.00446.x.

And on the reverse, we would have to believe that every marriage is a happily ever after, like in the movies. I'm sure we can think of people right now who are unhappily partnered or married.

So how do we shift away from the scarlet *S* of singledom? We learn to live our best lives.

In the following chapters, we will discuss how to reframe our perceptions and unlearn misconceptions, so that we aren't judging ourselves and our lives through that same harsh societal lens—and we'll learn practical ways to support our new empowered mentality!

CHAPTER 1:
RETHINKING SINGLE LIFE

Learning how to have fulfilling sexual encounters as a single person—whether engaging with brand new partners or relying on self-love to meet your needs—starts with learning to live a fulfilled single life in general. To achieve satisfying sexual encounters as single people, we first need to lay the foundations that will allow us to feel embodied and solid in our own single skin. The more empowered we feel in our daily lives, the more empowered we'll feel in sexual situations. So here in the early chapters of this book, we'll discuss ways to build those foundations by reducing stress, improving body image, and broadening our strategies for getting our needs met.

HOW TO NOT LEAD A FULFILLING SINGLE LIFE

Before we discuss how we singles can begin to reframe our experiences, overcome societal judgments, and learn to find joy in our current situations, let's take a look at some of the most common ways in which singles often undermine their own happiness and power. It's okay if you find yourself nodding your head in agreement with some of these behaviors. This isn't to call you out! It's to shine a light on the patterns you've been living with, and to teach you how to shift out of them and unlock the happiness you deserve.

Compare Yourself to Others

There's a well-known saying, commonly attributed to Theodore Roosevelt, that "Comparison is the thief of joy," and that couldn't be truer. If you think you've fallen behind your peer group, lamenting that you don't have a life like Stephanie's, you're going to make yourself miserable. Everyone's journey looks different, and there is no set timeline for when life events have to happen.

Worry About *Your* Timeline

"When is it going to happen to meee?!" I'm sure many of us had a preconceived idea of how our life would turn out. I really think it started with all of those MASH games we played on the playground. Truth be told, I'm glad I'm not living in a shack with Michael B, our nine kids, and a truck.

Should is a really loaded word. We can have an idea in our mind of how things "should" be, but ultimately, our own timeline unfolds at its own pace. I feel like there is so much pressure to have everything figured out by the time you're twenty-five, and that is so unrealistic. The fear of aging touches aspects beyond dating, prompting questions like: Will I still be attractive? Will my eggs still be good? What about my sex drive? Omg is that a grey hair?!

As you try to appreciate what you have here and now, you always have to keep this in the front of your mind: Someone else's journey is not yours. Their timeline has its own pace, with its own ups and downs. You can look at them for inspiration, but their timeline doesn't make your timeline less valid or important. There are no "shoulds" when it comes to relationships.

Obsess Over What Could Go Wrong

Hey! Stop that. Start to think about what you're able to control and what you're not. Constantly wondering if things are about to fall to shit can put a damper on your mental state. Always being on edge, waiting for the shoe to drop, can also be a self-fulfilling prophecy. You have to take things as they come, because you won't always get to choose how they come.

Expect Everything and Give Nothing

We aren't owed anything in this life. We are what we make of our lives. I am a firm believer in the idea that what you put out, you get back. If you do good, good will come back to you.

SELF-DECLARATION: HEAR ME ROAR

The world likes to put people into neat little rows, designations, and categories. Even though those descriptors may not be accurate representations of how you see yourself, society at large will classify you whether you like it or not. Sure, many of these labels aren't inherently bad, but there are some that can be limiting, demeaning, or harmful. For many, single is a glaring label that is often at the forefront of their description. Is that how you want to be viewed first?

Grab a piece of paper and write down who you are with the labels of your choice. Then, write down the labels that society has placed on you.

Don't know where to begin? Write down how your best friend would describe you. Thinking about yourself from their point of view can help you avoid the self-critical bias that we all carry and help you craft a more accurate and thoughtful description.

Compare your self-identified labels to what society "thinks" of you. Do they differ? Is there anything unexpected?

The important thing to remember is that you get to define who you are. Your self-identified labels are the ones that matter. Over time, as you keep expressing the truth of who you are and how the world should see you, others will follow your lead. This exercise can be repeated as you go through different seasons in life. Note how some things change and some things stay the same.

FREEDOMS AS A SINGLE PERSON

There are many benefits to being single, but one of the most highly valued benefits is the innate freedom that comes with this lifestyle. So, as you start to rethink your single life, appreciating the many freedoms you enjoy is a great way to start!

Flirt with abandon: As a single person, you have the opportunity to flirt whenever the chance arises. Especially if it's reciprocated, a little flirting can boost your confidence or be the gateway to something more.

Save money: You don't have to spend money on anyone but you! Or on you and your children, if you have kids. Also, you don't have to check in with anyone else about that big purchase you want to make.

Self-reliant: You can build a resiliency that might not have been available to you if you were partnered. Maybe you learn a new skill, like changing a sink faucet!

Sleep across the entire bed: I mean, is this not one of life's little pleasures? You aren't relegated to one side of the bed. This totally does not apply if you share your bed with a dog because you know that you get a sliver while they get the main share.

In a related benefit, you don't have to listen to anyone snoring in your ear at night. (Same canine exception applies.)

Wild nights: When was the last time you raged all night and didn't have to worry about being home by a certain time? Or what if the urge to bake bread struck you at 11:00 p.m.? You can do both and more! You don't have to worry about hurting someone's feelings or waking someone up with your kitchen activities.

You own the remote: You never have to compromise on what you want to watch.

First dates: You get to experience first dates! While this might not seem like a benefit, who doesn't love a little mystery? Even if it turns out to just be a nice date and not a relationship that progresses any further, first dates are filled with possibility!

Journal prompt: Why are you happy you're single? Why are you unhappy you're single?

FRIENDSHIPS AND BOUNDARIES

Just because we're single does not mean that we traverse this life alone. Family and friends are just as important as romantic partners. Friends and family can provide the amazing companionship, support, love, and adventure that you may not currently have with a partner. In fact, single people have the time and freedom to invest deeply in their relationships with their friends and family, meaning that these bonds can be incredibly strong. So whenever you feel alone, remember to recognize all that you have in terms of quality relationships already.

But as you take stock of your friendships, remember that it is important that you're surrounding yourself with people who build you up. Sometimes we can seem like easy targets because we are "alone," and people feel free to treat us in a harsher way. Here are some things to watch out for if you find yourself shying away from your support system.

Are you not receiving support from your current group of friends? Do you find yourself dreading an event or night out with them, always thinking of creative excuses to not go? Do you feel drained after being with them? Do you find the relationships to be one-sided—as if you're putting in more energy and effort than you ever get back? You may need some new friends!

Friendship is a special bond. These people become your tribe, your home team, and your family. They are there to support you during tough times and serve you real talk when you're being silly. While I don't think you need to keep a tally of who did what for whom, there needs to be an equitable exchange of support. Just because you are the single friend doesn't mean that you can drop everything to go to them.

Sometimes friends can be energy vampires and completely suck the life out of us. We cannot constantly build them up without some sort of reciprocation. Consider speaking up about this issue if you see it in your current friendships. It may be time to set some hard boundaries in terms of your time, your energy, or your space. You get to say how much you are willing to emotionally invest in a relationship. Whether you explicitly communicate those boundaries or just get in the habit of speaking up for yourself and your needs in the moment, setting up boundaries can save a friendship. Just like Robert Frost said, "Good fences make good neighbors."[6]

Another interesting sign to look for is growth. People change over time, as they gain more life experiences. Much like a romantic partner, everything in the beginning may have aligned well, but if there comes a time when you two are growing in different directions and cannot find common ground, it may be time for an end.

All endings do not have to be terrible. And just because something ended, that doesn't discount the value of what it was while it lasted. When the TV show *Breaking Bad* ended, of course I was sad, but I cherish it for what it was. There were good times, and I know there will be more (television shows) ahead for me in the future.

Your friends should be that group that you can go to for anything. They enrich your life, keep you accountable, and hold judgment-free space for you. If you find yourself starting to have trepidation about hanging out with them, ask

---

6 Robert Frost, "Mending Wall," *North of Boston* (David Nutt, 1914), https://www.poetryfoundation.org/poems/44266/mending-wall.

yourself why, and then address it with them. This isn't to say friendships should be conflict free—like anything that requires two people, problems and concerns arise. But with communication, clarity can often be found.

Remember, the only people who get upset when you have boundaries are the ones who benefitted when you had none.

Journal prompt: Have you ever had to end a friendship? Why? Looking back on it, do you feel you made the right choice?

STAYCATION

What can you tell me about the town you live in? Have you lived there all of your life, or are you a new transplant? If I were to come visit you, what would you tell me to do? Have you seen everything your area has to offer? Chances are you haven't. Take an outside view of where you call home and be a tourist in your own city. This is a fun activity to get you out of the house and open yourself up to positive interactions.

Go exploring. Do you have a tried-and-true favorite park trail that you like to walk on? Pull up your city's map and scope out some new territory. Seeing new sights and experiencing new environments can activate the imagination center of your mind. What would it be like if you lived closer to this park? What would happen if you took the left path as opposed to the right? Go find a different adventure!

Try a new restaurant. It's never been more popular to support local restaurants, so why not explore some new options? Your next favorite spot could be waiting for you to pop in and enjoy their offerings. If you're going to be dining alone, ask to sit at the bar and poll the staff on their favorite menu picks. Also, this activity is great with a friend because you can sample double the amount of food.

Utilize the internet. Thanks to technology (and COVID-19), there is literally something going on at any time of the day or night online. You already know what you like, so why not try something different? Join a group for neighborhood clean-up or attend a Zoom class on how to make pasta. There are so many cool activities out there, you're bound to find one you like. And if your experiment is a total bust, at least it will make a great story later.

Cities are always growing and expanding, so there's always something new to discover. And with your freedom as a single person, adventure is right around the corner. Be brave and branch out. I know you can do it!

SOLO TRAVEL

Solo-cation? Sign me up! A vacation is a wonderful way to reset physically, mentally, and spiritually. As a single person, you don't have to coordinate with someone else's schedule or ask permission—you're the captain now.

You are the activities directory of your solo vacation, and you can do whatever you want, on whatever schedule suits you. If you want to go on the chocolate factory tour, go do it! If you want to book the medicinal plant and foraging class, you can! If you want to rent the swan paddle boat and paddle with the other couples, get to pumping those legs! Plan your ideal itinerary, with the surety that no one will object.

Researching, planning, and scheduling your trip can make you feel like a boss. And while you're exploring, it's likely you'll make new friends along the way! Maybe when you're scuba diving, you'll get partnered with someone you get along well with, and then boom—instant friendship. Don't be surprised if a close connection forms based on exciting shared memories.

You don't have to break the bank when it comes to vacationing. What might you explore in the next town over? Just get out there and participate in activities you wouldn't usually try.

Journal prompt: Research a dream destination and plan your lodging, activities, and must-see attractions. Save for future use!

MAKING YOUR DREAMS COME TRUE

Manifesting is about making your dreams into a reality. It's wonderful to have big dreams, but how to go about achieving that end result may not be so clear. Here are some steps to help you on your journey.

Determine your goal. We need to know what we're striving for. Writing your goal down in a visible location keeps it front of mind and gives it permanence.

Embrace gratitude. Before you embark on manifesting a new goal, look back to where you started. Recognize all that has come to you already. By keeping gratitude as the attitude, you will be attracting more and more of what you want into your life.

Be active. You have to do more than just think yourself to success. You have to be an active participant by ensuring the choices you make day by day are helping move you closer to your goal.

Trust the process. Manifestation isn't something that happens overnight, so stay the course and continue to believe that you're moving closer to your goal with each effort.

Stay upbeat. Everyone falters from time to time, but remember that whatever is meant for you is already on its way to you. Resilience is the key to achieving your dreams.

Journal prompt: If you had a magic wand, what would you gift yourself? What steps can you take now to make that gift a reality?

Making Personal Goals

This is such an overlooked aspect of being single. The world is literally at your fingertips, and you can do just about anything. Make some goals! Learn how to cook a foreign cuisine. Read! Schedule out time for meditation. Sign up to volunteer somewhere. Actually hang your laundry in the closet instead of searching through the three baskets on the floor. These activities and more are great things to work toward. You can make these goals as big or as small as you'd like, there are really no limitations. As a single person, you are more likely to have the time to better yourself and continue growing by crushing goals.

Say Yes

If you don't have children, then you are a party of one, so saying yes to invitations should be fairly easy. You don't need to coordinate with your partner's schedule or see if the babysitter is free. Even if something sounds weird, try it. By keeping your life open to opportunity, you are increasing your chance for adventure and networking. Single and confident people are out there! They are pursuing passions and smashing fears.

I JUST DONT LIKE BEING SINGLE

I hear you. Trying to deny sadness around anything is never a good idea. It is absolutely okay to feel sad about not being in a relationship. Wanting more intimacy, companionship, and partnership is a valid desire. Our lives are full of sadness around "wanting." You waited in line for fifteen minutes only to learn that your favorite ice cream was sold out (I love you blueberry cobbler ice cream!), and you had to wait until they had it again. Of course this is a simplification, but it doesn't mean that it's a poor example of being sad about something you can't have right now.

But you can acknowledge the feelings, and then make a decision to make the best of the situation. Insert lemon soft serve.

What are you in control of? Many aspects of your life are within your control. You can decide how to set the thermostat in your house, whether or not you want to eat ice cream straight from the container, or if you want to cut your hair off.

Of course, when it comes to relationships, we're looking at two variables. One of those variables is you. The other is someone else. You cannot control the feelings, actions, or desires of another person. If something is beyond your control, release your hold on it. I know I just got a blowout and now it's raining—I can't control the weather, just like I can't control my curls from coming back.

Acknowledge your sadness over being single, but don't dwell on it. Life is forever changing, and your romantic relationship (or lack thereof) is only one aspect of your full and vibrant life. This is why I love having a gratitude list (and where journaling can be your friend). Look at all of the positives you have going on in your life, and then ask yourself if being single is the worst thing you can be. Even if it takes you a while to come up with a list, I know there are things that you have that others wish they could have. Once you can reframe your outlook, it can help give you perspective on the hierarchy of importance when it comes to your dating life.

Do not let fear drive you into an ill-fitting relationship. "At least I'm not alone" is never a great reason to be in a relationship. A partner will not be able to solve all of your problems, concerns, or needs. This becomes more glaringly true when it isn't the right person from the start.

If you feel this disappointment as a constant, reach out to family and friends and let them know you're struggling. Another idea to help give you some perspective is volunteering with a helping organization. While you absolutely cannot work from an empty cup, try to see what filling others' cups feels like. It may help you to see that your cup wasn't as empty as you thought it was. Giving back also feels good, and it can help boost your sense of connection.

Remember, just because it hasn't happened yet doesn't mean that it never will. Trust the path!

Journal Prompt: What facets about singledom are keeping you up at night? Sometimes putting distressing things to paper can help lessen their hold on our contentment.

HOW TO BE A THIRD WHEEL

Being a third wheel often has a negative connotation, but I'd like to shift this definition. If we see being a third wheel as a couple taking pity on their single friend, of course it's going to sound bad. But if we make it into something positive, then the third wheel might become the next cool thing! Maybe. Too much wishful thinking?

First of all, let's look at the facts. You have two friends! Hurray! That's awesome, we're already starting out at a high. If they invited you out, they want to see you and they enjoy your company.

Keep the reminders that you're single to a minimum with them. They know. If you start to lament your single status every time you see them do something couple-y (think PDA), it will likely make all of you feel uncomfortable.

Great third wheels know that they can be the unofficial photographer for the evening. Short of asking the server for a photo, how often do couples have the opportunity to have their photos taken without it being a selfie? Give back to your friends. Bonus: you can always snap a photo of yourself with them kissing in the background to let everyone know you're on a date, sort of.

Being a third wheel can also give you insights for your future relationship. You get an insider's glimpse into what is and isn't working in your friends' relationship. All of that information can be stored away for future use. And don't forget, if they have kids, you get to have the wonderful title of aunt or uncle.

LOVE SINGLE LIFE—MISS TOUCH

Spontaneously baking bread at 11:00 p.m., deciding to go

on a spur-of-the-moment trip, and saying yes to last-minute theater tickets are just a few of the innumerable things that single people have the freedom to indulge in. Even with this wide breadth of opportunity, there are a few things that are inescapable for the single person, and one of them is missing physical touch. Physical touch is often taken for granted, but when absent from a life, it can become glaringly obvious. Missing touch is a completely normal experience. We are not meant to traverse this life without it.

How to Cultivate Sensuality

Feeling sensual doesn't have to be some big production—we don't need a lot of external props. We can experience the sensuality in our daily lives. When you're feeling off, it helps to strip everything away and get back into basics.

What can you feel with your body? Considering we spend up to half of our lives in bed, is it time that you upgraded your sheets? In a study conducted by Slumber Cloud,[7] they found that 75 percent of people said their bed could be more comfortable. My editor at the first magazine I ever wrote for said, "Always splurge on your sheets." I've taken that to heart ever since. If this is supposed to be your place of rest, why stock it with less than luxurious fabrics?

Speaking of bedding, have you considered a weighted blanket? These have been all the rage lately, as they can provide some powerful relief when it comes to anxiety and restlessness. They have been used to treat conditions like

---

7 Kate Mellot, "How To Build a Bedder Relationship with Your Bed," Slumber Cloud, last modified March 21, 2019, https://www.slumbercloud.com/blog/better-relationship-with-your-bed/.

anxiety and autism. Their comforting weight feels like a hug and can be just the tactile thing you need to upgrade your quality of sleep.

What can you smell or taste? There's nothing like the smell or taste of a particular food to return you to a fond memory. Consider adding ingredients you really enjoy into your pantry and taking the time to savor your meals. If you're a kitchen person, take your time smelling and tasting the ingredients as you craft something from your heart, for your stomach.

Sometimes we need to restart, and a shower can be the perfect vehicle to return us to ourselves. Really notice the sensations of the water moving over your body, and take time to lather yourself up. Consider purchasing some fresh eucalyptus to hang in your shower for aroma therapy. Essential oils like lavender and eucalyptus can also be sprinkled on the floor, to become more pungent as the hot water steam infuses the bathroom with their scent.

If you're by yourself and you want to feel embodied, consider dancing. Put on your favorite music and move in a way that makes your body feel good. Hopping and bopping around can boost your mood and help you revel in gratitude for all of the things your body is able to do.

To tap into our sensuality, sometimes we need a little guidance. There are many guided meditations online that can help put you in a mindset in which you'll more readily feel and notice all of the sensations around you. I'm personally a fan of the Calm app, which offers resources for better sleep, relaxation, and meditation.[8]

---

8 Calm, v. 5.11 (Calm.com, Inc., 2012).

Some people also find *grounding* to be beneficial, as a way to bring them back to themselves. Grounding is the technique of making connections with the earth. Walking barefoot, for instance, can help you connect to the earth's electrons and can boost your health. In the *Journal of Environmental and Public Health*, one study found evidence of its subjects having an increased satisfaction with sleep quality and level of restfulness after grounding, in comparison to their control counterparts.[9]

Sensuality is available in so many aspects of our lives already—we just have to know how to recognize it and relish in its existence.

SKIN HUNGER

Skin hunger is the basic, natural need for contact. And I'm talking about physical contact, so technology can't help us here. A meaningful touch. Something that can be hard to come by, especially when you're single. I know you might be thinking, "So what? I might go days without touch. It's not like I need it to survive," and you'd be right. Sort of.

While touch is not essential to keeping us alive, it's still essential for quality of life. This need has been documented by scientific studies. Harry Harlow was an American psychologist best known for his work with infant rhesus monkeys. If you'd like to view them, some clips of his experiments are on the internet. They're hard to watch. What was considered "controversial" back in his day is

---

9 Gaetan Chevalier et al., "Earthing: Health Implications of Reconnecting the Human Body to the Earth's Surface Electrons," *Journal of Environmental and Public Health* (January 12, 2012), https://doi.org/10.1155/2012/291541.

surely unethical today. I'll describe them here to save you from the visual trauma.

Harlow was researching the impact of physical touch when it came to rearing infant monkeys. More specifically, does touch play a role when it comes to development? His many experiments and inquiries on touch demonstrated that touch was an integral part of normal development. In one instance, when given the choice of a wire mom that provided food or a soft mom that gave them no food, the infant monkeys choose the soft mom, despite it not having food. The data was compelling and led him to surmise that touch is essential in the development and well-being of these monkeys. Those who were isolated without touch demonstrated severe developmental delays and behavioral issues. These issues grew worse with extended periods of no contact. So, long story short, extrapolated into human behavior, it only makes sense that we too seek out the comfort of touch for our well-being. Without enough physical touch, we might start experiencing issues like depression and anxiety.[10]

As a single person, you may not have the option of sharing skin with someone on the regular. You don't need a partner to have touch in your life, though. There are many options out there to help you feed the hunger.

Masturbation: Be Your Own Best Lover

Superstitions abound when it comes to masturbation! Your genitals will fall off, you'll waste all of your semen, you'll

---

10 Kory Floyd, "Relational and Health Correlates of Affection Deprivation," *Western Journal of Communication* 78, no. 4 (July 15, 2014): 383–403, https://doi.org/https://doi.org/10.1080/10570314.2014.927071.

become a sex addict—these are all myths when it comes to self-love. The superstitions still persist in our society, so if you've never touched yourself, you're not alone. Along with those fears, many people have guilt and shame around masturbation. These ideas are usually formed during our childhood and teenage years and stay with us through adulthood.

Taps microphone Masturbation is normal and completely healthy! Consider this your permission slip to explore your body and receive pleasure.

Need some more convincing? Masturbation is one of the 100% safe sexual activities you can do that have no risk of STI transmission or pregnancy. Engaging in self-love is also an easy and free way to help alleviate stress. Its healing properties have been known to relieve cramps and even help you sleep better. With the release of the feel-good endorphins produced by masturbation, you'll be on your way to a lovely afterglow sleep in no time.

Touching yourself is a wonderful way to get in touch with your body and discover that your next lover is only one hand slide away. The more you get to know your body, the better you will be able to communicate your preferences to future partners. And keep in mind that masturbation is not some last choice activity out of desperation. Masturbation can absolutely be the main course, so stop thinking of it as three-day-old pizza in the fridge (which arguably can still be quite good). More on this later.

Friend Relationships
A friend is a safe option when seeking out platonic touch. Clearly consent is needed first, but don't discount this already cultivated relationship. As long as they're willing, you can

both reap the rewards. Although, it's a good idea to have a conversation around boundaries before you begin.

Cuddling with a friend gives you the benefits of physical touch, plus it's a chance to hang out with your friend! The kids call that a win-win situation.

In fact, hugging for at least twenty seconds has been shown to have measurable health benefits. In a study done at the University of North Carolina at Chapel Hill, researchers concluded that higher oxytocin levels and lower blood pressure resulted from a twenty-second hug between partners.[11] Think about all of the hugs you could be cashing in on.

Just remember, let your friends know what's up before you latch on like a baby koala. This is for my health! Love me!

Pets

Otherwise known as earth angels, pets are simply the best, and their worth is only bolstered by the health benefits they provide. They enrich our lives in myriad ways, but snuggling them is top of the list. When you cuddle your pet, you both benefit from the mutual release of oxytocin, which can help strengthen the connection you two share. Several animal studies lend support to this idea as well. One study showed that oxytocin was increased when rats had their bellies rubbed.[12] I mean, same. Just another outlet to feed the hunger with.

---

11 Karen M. Grewen, et al., "Warm Partner Contact Is Related to Lower Cardiovascular Reactivity," *Behavioral Medicine* 29, no. 3 (March 25, 2010): 123–130, https://doi. org/https://doi.org/10.1080/08964280309596065.

12 Moberg, et al., "Self-soothing behaviors with particular reference to oxytocin release induced by non-noxious sensory stimulation." *Frontiers in Psychology* 5, no. 1529 (January 12, 2015), https://doi.org/10.3389/fpsyg.2014.01529.

Hire a Professional

Is this in the White Pages under the letter "C"? (Wait, did I just date myself by writing "White Pages"? It's what we had before Google.) Cuddle Buddy is a job you probably didn't see on career day, but this growing practice is one in which you can hire a certified professional whose job is to snuggle with you.

How does it work? There are codes of conduct to keep everyone comfortable and maintain safe boundaries. Make sure you're asking lots of questions from a potential cuddle buddy. Seek out recommendations and look into their service background so that you know you aren't being hoodwinked into snuggling a rogue person. It might seem weird, but these professionals are providing a valuable service that is unavailable to many people. Sure, you may not be willing to publicly check in to the "Cuddle Center" on Facebook, but don't discount this viable option.

Over the ten years from 2007 to 2017, "the share of U.S. adults living without a spouse or partner . . . climbed to 42%, up from 39%," according to a Pew Research Center article.[13] We can only infer that the amount of touch in the lives of US adults will be even less now, with the prevalence of all the digital interactions we rely on, particularly after the COVID-19 pandemic made digital connection more popular. Even less opportunity for touching. There are some things that even Amazon Prime can't deliver you.

---

13 Richard Fry, "The Share of Americans Living without a Partner Has Increased, Especially among Young Adults," Pew Research Center, last modified October 11, 2017, https://www.pewresearch.org/fact-tank/2017/10/11/the-share-of-americans

PHONE SEX ANECDOTE

Sometimes when physical avenues of connection are unavailable to us, people opt to use technology. There are chatrooms, message boards, and even phone sex operators to help us stay connected with others. In fact, I was once a phone sex operator.

I remember one summer, stay-at-home moms were making news by paying for their family vacations by doing phone sex. I was intrigued. The only experience I had with phone sex was watching depictions in TV or movies. I needed to find out what it was really like. I found a company that was hiring, and after a short interview, I was in! This of course meant I had to go out and buy a corded telephone. Let me tell you, that was quite the experience in and of itself. I called my phone provider and asked to have a landline activated—another weird experience, but easily done. I was set and ready to go!

Not to spoil the ending, but my phone sex career lasted ten days. I kept saying this would make a great chapter in my book, and well, here we are. I remember being nervous about my first call. What would it be like? Would I have to initiate the conversation? So many questions. We communicated with our dispatch operators by instant messenger. They would let us know who the caller was (if it was a repeat customer), what they were looking for, and what kind of session they had paid for. Customers were broken down into people who had prepaid for a set amount of time, those who paid by the minute, or those who had a set time with the option to expand their time.

My first caller was ready. He was on the pay per minute plan and was eager to go. I can't remember what was said as we began, but I will never forget what happened at the end. After building him up and telling him his was the biggest and best penis I'd ever had (I was really good with the voices), he began to come. Long mooooan, groan, fast breathing, and then CLICK. I honestly pulled the phone away from my ear and looked at the receiver. I was shocked! He didn't even say goodbye!

I learned that many customers didn't say goodbye once they'd received what they called for. The only other standout call I had was when a caller was very drunk. It was after 2:00 a.m., and it was a prime time to be available. This was a new caller I had never spoken to before. He had chosen the prepay option for a set amount of time. I answered using my sweet phone sex voice, and he was instantly aggressive and rude. If anyone spoke to me like that in real life, we would have had problems, but I was phone sex babe and I rolled with it. At one point he stopped responding to me, and I stopped talking to listen. He had fallen asleep and was snoring on the open line.

I thought it was perfect karma to leave him on the line while he snoozed, and I painted my nails. At the end of our allotted time, I said thanks and hung up. I'd like to believe that he had a shocking charge amount the next time his credit card bill came due. Moral of the story, however you search for connection, always be nice.

CHAPTER:2
SELF-CARE

Ordinarily, I'd say that there is a fair amount of stress in our lives, but with COVID-19 turning 2020 on its head, stress in America went significantly up for the first time since polling began in 2007, according to the American Psychological Association. The average reported stress level (on a scale of 1–10) for US adults was 4.9 back in 2019, but for 2020 was 5.4 (COVID-19–related stress alone ranked at 5.9).[14]

With that being said, stress is a robust factor that can impact your sexuality. Whether it affects your energy, desire, or how you feel about yourself, this is one we have to address up front. If we can help mitigate the stress in your life—because it will never fully go away—we can start to create a plan that lets you move through life without having to reach the burnout stage. Also, if you've found effective ways to manage your stress, it will help you be better able to receive and implement the advice in the rest of this book!

14 "Stress in the Time of COVID-19, Volume One," American Psychological Association, last modified May 2020, https://www.apa.org/news/press/releases/stress/2020/report.

SELF-CARE BASICS

Come most Januarys, many of us find ourselves resolving to make a great change, fueled by the "new year, new you" enthusiasm. I'm here to tell you that you do not have to make a bargain with yourself to make a change. And there certainly isn't a limitation on when you can start.

When thinking about making changes to your life, remember first and foremost that you are fantastic, amazing, and great already! Instead of looking for flaws or negatives about yourself, look at the positives, and think of what could make your life even more wonderful. Being mindful of how strong and beautiful you are is important.

Take an inventory of what's going on in your life right now. List below what sort of things stress you out, and what is giving you joy.

_____

_____

_____

_____

_____

_____

Maybe you've written down items like school, having a job, relationships, family, friends, finances, or the future. These big-picture variables will likely not be going anywhere in your life anytime soon. These will be constants—sometimes more prominent than at other times, but you will never be without them. So once we can account for the constants, let's look at how the variables available to us can help us create a life that we don't feel like we need to escape from.

Answer these true/false statements for yourself:

I have enough time to devote to family and friends.
I have time to eat healthy most days.
I often have enough time in the day scheduled for "me time."
Most of the time, I am not stressed.
I have enough time to spend on things I love to do.
I feel energized and well rested most of the time.
I never have a hard time saying no.
I rarely have trouble sleeping.
I am not easily angered or agitated.
I have enough time in my day to move my body in ways I enjoy.

Take stock of your results. Are you pleased with how many times you said true? Was this exercise dominated by many false responses? Whatever the case may be, you can always change your lifestyle to make those false responses become your truth. You can always improve your self-care to help prevent becoming overwhelmed—aka: chill out before you burn out.

Sometimes our lives can feel like they're spiraling out of control, but you can act now! Start today to make yourself a priority.

People commonly mistake self-care as selfish. We have been indoctrinated into a society that says "More is more!" and leaves little room for saying no without a heaping load of guilt. I hope I'm not the first person to say this to you, but if I am, consider me saying each word punctuated with the clapping of my hands: Self. Care. Isn't. Just. Important. It's. Crucial!

I'll say it again, for the people in the back. Self-care isn't just important; it's crucial. We have to shift from the mindset that saying yes to more, and sacrificing our time and emotional resources, will bring us greater joy or achievement in the end. There is no prize for burning ourselves out.

And here's the thing about self-care: It isn't just bath bombs and brunch. Sometimes it can look as foundational as getting up to take a shower. While some self-care options can be luxurious, it doesn't necessarily mean that all self-care is luxury. I love freshly baked chocolate chip cookies and a massage as much as the next person, but those aren't items that are topping the chart of my self-care list. For me, things like drinking water, eating nourishing food, getting outdoors, and playing with my dogs help keep me on a fairly level path to avoid burnout.

Self-neglect, even though that sounds like an ugly phrase, is so easy to slip into, especially if we're busy. Even taking a small break can feel forbidden, despite our mind and body desperately sending us the signals that we need to slow down. We learn to push these cues away, and only when they pile up do they finally manifest themselves in negative ways.

WHAT CAN BURNOUT LOOK LIKE?

For those who may not relate to what I've been saying, or those who have further questions on what exactly burnout looks like, consider these your signs:

Reduced performance: And I don't mean like you-just-finished-a-marathon exhausted. You find yourself tired from your daily routine. Your creativity may be lacking, or you just have no more zest for doing your work. You may even feel resentful about it.

You don't feel good: Things like frequent stomachaches, headaches, or other physical manifestations can also be a sign of burnout.

Emotional exhaustion: You're feeling overwhelmed and unable to cope with your current situation. You're lacking the motivation to get your list of daily things done, and you have trouble concentrating.

Some of these symptoms are also shared with mental health conditions like depression. If you're feeling a sense of hopelessness about your life, please seek out help. If you're having suicidal thoughts, please contact the National Suicide Prevention Lifeline. There is help for you.

If left unaddressed, burnout can lead to depression, or to unhealthy coping mechanisms. We want to be proactive and help create a life that you don't have to escape from.

So, how do we do self-care? Start small! Make changes that are simple and easily attainable. Many small promises to yourself are easy to achieve, as opposed to major lifestyle changes. Then, when you do them, celebrate! Often we are looking for a gigantic payoff in the end, and we forget to celebrate the small accomplishments along the way. Consider what goals you are looking to implement into your self-care routine.

And once you have your self-care routine down, protect your schedule. This can mean saying no to things, which can be hard, but remember, we are starting to place ourselves first.

Another aspect of self-care that many people struggle with, especially when undertaking a large lifestyle change, is guilt. So you completely skipped the gym this week or you ended up eating two pieces of pie. Bring on the shame shower. Stop! Do not get discouraged if you stumble from your path.

I've heard women, myself included, saying "I have to be good" in response to something they want to do, as a reminder that they shouldn't be doing what is offered to them. What about being good to yourself? Is that one day of drinking wine with the girls or that one week of skipping yoga going to shatter your dreams of achieving your goal? I hope not. Each day is a new one, so start it as such.

We need to have forgiveness worked into our self-care plan. So while you are finding out what is right for you and trying your best to stick to that, it's okay if you stumble.

BEFORE THE BAD DAY PLAN

No one wakes up planning a bad day. Bad days pop up unexpectedly in our lives and their duration can vary. Today (like, right now) I want you to set yourself up for success and equip yourself with a list of things that bring you joy. Why make this list now, on a (presumably) good day? If you're in the midst of a difficult time, you're not likely to want to attempt my exercise, and then you'll be caught without a plan for stopping the downward spiral. Try to make this a physical list and put it somewhere that you can see it easily.

Think of both budget-friendly and splurge activities.

Here are some examples:

- ▸ Read a book for pleasure. Stop looking at your screen and let your eyes take you on a journey.
- ▸ Get outside. Ditch the technology and take in some

fresh air. Changing your environment can also have a positive impact on your mood, so step outdoors and breathe deeply.

▸ Write about gratitude. Take some deep breaths and write down the positive aspects of your life. Even if times seem bleak, seeing how much good you have in your life can help reframe whatever has you feeling down.

▸ Take a long shower or bath. Let the healing power of water soothe your body and wash away your troubles. Really luxuriate in the feeling of the water against your skin.

▸ When in doubt, masturbate. This is the ultimate near-cure-all that you have in your bag of tricks. Touching your body can take your mind off whatever's ruining your day and release a wave of feel-good hormones. Orgasm doesn't have to be the goal, but it can be a great side effect!

Once you've made your list, you can pick a few things to try the next time you're having a bad day, and you'll immediately be on the path to healing. Don't restrict yourself to just the activities on the list, if you come up with new ideas. You can also format your plan to include reminders of supportive people in your life and your overall self-care goals. Here's an example worksheet that you can use for your bad day plan.

SELF-CARE PLAN

SexologistMegan.com (c) 2019

PEOPLE WHO SUPPORT ME

- ACTIVITIES THAT ARE -

	HELPFUL	HARMFUL
MIND		
BODY		
SPIRIT		

I WANT TO ACCOMPLISH

TIPS FOR SETTING SELF-CARE GOALS

Making goals is a great way to consistently work on your self-care plan. Here are some things to consider when setting up your list:

Be realistic about your own schedule: Don't set yourself up for failure by saying that you'll go to the gym five times a week if you're working two jobs. That just seems unrealistic.

Start small and work your way up: Don't tell yourself that you're going to drink at least three liters of water every day for a month.[15] You could totally do that, but what if you don't complete your task for a few days? Will you feel empowered? Not likely—you'll probably feel defeated. Maybe you can say that you'll drink three liters at least two times a week.

Think consistency: Is this goal something that you will be able to do consistently? If it's too big, reframe it until it's something that can be easily worked into your daily schedule.

Prioritize: How do you rank these goals that you've set for yourself? Are they important enough to warrant space in your daily routine? If so, make sure you give them the attention they deserve.

---

15 Opinions vary on the appropriate amount of water to drink per day. Your hydration needs will depend on many factors, including your gender, diet, activity level, health conditions, and age. Drinking too much water can be detrimental to those with particular health concerns. Consult a doctor before drastically increasing your intake.

Think short term and long term: Some goals may only have a short-term window, and others might be lifelong pursuits. Your goal for getting more water in your life might be a lifelong challenge, but the goal of waking up early to do yoga in the mornings might just last while you're in school.

Making and Tracking Specific Objectives

In order to track goals effectively, you should try to use the following framework.

When writing down your self-care objectives:

▸ Be concise.
▸ Use "I statements" ("I will _____.").
▸ Be as specific as possible.

Once you've set your objectives, here are some tips to help you stay on track:

▸ Track your progress. Find a solution that works for you. You already know how much I love my bullet journal. You can have a nightly check-in where you write about what you did that day and how it affected your mood—making note of what works and what doesn't. If you're still having resistance to journaling, feel free to at least talk it out in your mind so you can try to pinpoint the best plan of action. You could also try using a color-coded calendar. Whatever system feels sustainable for you, and whatever will help you get into a routine.

▸ Make a checklist. It's very satisfying to check off a completed task. And let's be real here, I can't be the only one who writes down already completed tasks just to check them off again right?

▶ Recognize achievements. Celebrate your wins, yo! Not everything you do has to be some grand thing. A little win goes a long way. And forgive yourself when you stumble.

You are the creator of your goals, so why not set yourself up for success! There is plenty of room for adjustment and change as different factors move in and out of your life like workload, relationships, and health.

SQUARE BREATHING EXERCISE

If ever you find yourself in a place where you just-need-five-minutes-of-peace-okay?!, try square breathing. Ideally this is done in a peaceful place, but you can utilize this anywhere and any time you need to reset yourself with the power of breath.

▶ Step 1. Slowly exhale all of your air.
▶ Step 2. Gently inhale through your nose for a four count.
▶ Step 3. Hold at the top of your inhale for a four count.
▶ Step 4. Gently exhale through your mouth for a four count.
▶ Step 5. Hold empty for a four count.
▶ Step 6. Repeat.

It can be helpful to visualize a square as you do this. There are also gifs and animations you can search online to help you with this, if it's challenging to keep track with your mind.

Also, if you're in a hurry and need a shot of relaxation, take a big deep belly breath and audibly exhale it through your mouth. By doing this, you are indirectly stimulating the vagus nerve. These deep breaths activate neurons that signal the vagus nerve that our blood pressure is becoming too high, and it responds by lowering our heart rate. Thanks science! Give it a try now!

Big breath in!
Audible exhale!

Big breath in!
Audible exhale!

How do you feel now?

DAILY GRATITUDE CHECK-IN

As I've mentioned, journaling can be a great tool to help you get an overview of how your life is going over time. While keeping your eye on the prize, you can sometimes overlook, or discount, the daily joys of living. Yes, having an end goal is productive, but don't forget to enjoy the journey there. Celebrate your little victories wherever they appear.

What is a little victory? Maybe you remembered to put the garbage out on the right day. Perhaps you hit your daily water consumption goal in your bullet journal. Or possibly you just had a really good day at work! It doesn't matter how grand or small, wins are piling up. Noticing the abundance of goodness happening around you can boost your overall mood and attitude. Be an active observer of life's joys and beauties. Perhaps you've never really noticed how much pleasure, bounty, and kindness is around you all of the time.

Journal prompt: Ask yourself the following questions before bed: What am I grateful for? What am I working toward? What do I hope tomorrow brings?

MOOD TRACKER

Tracking your mood in your journal is a great way to recognize any patterns you may be experiencing in life. Bullet journals are great for tracking your various moods and can be fun to fill out as the days go on. Or maybe analog isn't your style and you want to keep track via an app. Any solution that works for you is the right one!

Before you start coloring in a box or marking your mood in an app, sit back and reflect on what your day has been like. What was your stress level like? Did you get enough sleep? Did something noteworthy happen and impact your mood? The more detail you can give yourself the better. Then, mark down your mood. After a time, you'll be able to visually see any trends. Perhaps you were content and peaceful on those evenings after you visited your best friend. Maybe you found your brain spinning with anxiety at night whenever big deadlines were approaching. Over time you might start to correlate certain emotions with certain events or people. With that knowledge in hand, if something is on the horizon that you know will drain you, you can better plan around it and try to have a buffer afterwards to mitigate your feelings.

Tracking your mood can show you trends or help you pinpoint triggers. A trigger is a reminder of a past event that elicits a strong reaction. For example, maybe a song you liked played on the radio and then a little while later you started to feel down. The event itself wasn't noteworthy, you think—you just heard a song that you used to love. But maybe upon reflection, you realize that it was a song that you and your ex-partner used to listen to, and subconsciously it made you sad. Taking the time to note your mood and what influenced it can help you navigate emotional triggers in the future.

After journaling and tracking your mood for a while, try filling out the following worksheet, which is a handy quick guide. Post it somewhere visible, as you would with your "Bad Day Plan." This sort of worksheet can serve as a reminder of your proven self-care strategies and the best ones to turn to on a bad day.

NAME

PEOPLE IN MY CORNER

GOALS

THINGS I NEED
FOR SUCCESS

THINGS DETRIMENTAL
TO SUCCESS

SexologistMegan.com

Here's an example of how I filled out this worksheet:

NAME *Megan*

PEOPLE IN MY CORNER

Diane MaryLynne Jennie Kelsey Stephanie

GOALS

Finish writing my book

Make time for yoga

No more bad dates

THINGS I NEED FOR SUCCESS

Support when I'm feeling down. Leave the house to go work. Radical honestey. Saying no more often.

THINGS DETRIMENTAL TO SUCCESS

technology distractions. feeling lonely. not setting boundaries

SexologistMegan.com

After you've made charting your moods a daily habit, it can be useful, and sometimes inspiring, to reflect on the past emotional tone of your life. Your feelings may have been all over the place, and that's normal! It isn't a sign that you weren't working toward bettering yourself every day. Every new day is a chance to begin again and another opportunity to work on growth, happiness, and reaching your goals.

Once you're well into your charting journey, it can be cathartic to look back and see all of the progress you've made. Chances are that your feelings won't have been linear, but that doesn't mean that you've regressed. Each day forward is another step toward healing and building peace within your life. You may even find that you'll continue to chart your mood as part of your daily ritual. This can be a wonderful addition to your life.

EMOTIONAL BREAKDOWN EXERCISE

Even after you've set goals, cuddled with your pet, taken a solo vacation, and taught yourself how to cook bibimbap, you may find sadness or disappointment building up on you. This can be particularly likely in times of increased isolation and decreased opportunities for touch. From time to time, these intense emotions may hit you harder, and may even lead to what feels like an emotional breakdown.

Here is an exercise that can help you try to understand where your emotional breakdown is coming from.

- ▸ Ask yourself how you feel.
- ▸ Ask yourself why you might be feeling this way.
- ▸ Ask yourself how long you've been feeling this way.
- ▸ Ask yourself if you think this feeling will last.
- ▸ Ask yourself what you're going to do if this feeling doesn't go away.

Being able to piece apart your problem can help you understand the building blocks of your breakdown. Maybe this emotion will be fleeting, and you won't have to worry about it for much longer. Maybe this is something that will have a long-term impact on your life.

Repeating this exercise, even when times are good, can be a helpful exercise. Being able to chart your feelings and look back at where you've been can be very helpful in the healing process.

Journal prompt: Write about something you'd like to work on, emotionally. Write about something you'd like to grow through.

ROOM REFRESH

Have you ever considered the impact that your environment plays on your psyche and well-being? According to IKEA's Life At Home Report (2018), "1 in 3 people all over the world say there are places where they feel more at home than the space they live in."

The researchers see home as a multidimensional combination of place, space, things, and relationships. In their study, factors influencing people to not feel at home included: a lack of comfort, making some feel restricted; a sense of not belonging, making some feel disconnected with their space; and inadequate privacy, leading 23% of people to leave their house in order to have some alone time.

So how do we make our space feel like a home?

Feng shui, the practice of arranging your home in a way to best help you achieve your life goals, takes your environment into account very seriously. The overarching idea behind feng shui is that the major to micro things that comprise your space can either work with you or against you. By understanding how certain things can affect your life, you can better create a space that will help you thrive. Some purported benefits of arranging your home under the principles of feng shui include:

▶ Better sleep
▶ Increased motivation
▶ Improved health
▶ More active sex life
▶ More harmonious relationships
▶ Better relaxation at home
▶ Greater feeling of control

Take an online quiz to find out what your feng shui birth element is. I looked up mine and it was totally spot on! How do they know me?! Simple things like moving the position of your bed to a protected corner of your room can help with better sleep, and decluttering your space can facilitate better energy flow. For more on how to make your space work for you, consider checking out *The Life-Changing Magic of Tidying Up: The Japanese Art of Decluttering and Organizing* by Marie Kondo, or *A Master Course in Feng-Shui: An In-Depth Program for Learning to Choose, Design, and Enhance the Spaces Where We Live and Work* by Eva Wong.

Crystals

Some people find comfort in the use of healing crystals. The belief behind this practice is that various rocks are tangible connections to the earth. Each of them have their own unique vibration pattern that can help you on your path to healing. Placing them against your skin or in your environment is said to amplify your own thoughts and intentions. Different crystals help with different concerns, so look up which ones might best serve you in your space.

Scents

Scent is a powerful, and often overlooked, aspect of our environment. Scents have the ability to take us back to a certain place in our memories. Maybe it was a summer when we were young, maybe it reminds us of a specific family member? As far as using scent in our spaces, the research suggests that we can create a whole host of positive effects by just breathing. Numerous studies have cited the use of essential oils in helping relieve stress and pain. They can also help with improving mood and boosting cognitive function. For example, scents from the citrus family, like lemon and grapefruit, have been said to be energizing and to improve brain function.

Colors

Color is another impactful way to influence the space you live in. The way you feel around certain colors is very personal and drawn from your own life experiences. Ask yourself how you felt each year as Pantone released their color of the year. Did you love it? Did you immediately say no thank you? Color impacts us everywhere.

Chromatherapy is the use of visible light to heal your physical and spiritual body. The different colors have different vibratory properties, and all you need to do is sit in the color to treat whatever is ailing you. It has been practiced by many ancient cultures throughout time and is still prevalent in designing almost everything we consume. While cool colors like blues, greens, and purples have been commonly cited to produce calming effects, you may find another color soothing to you. Personally, I love shades of gray. And yes, it does stem from my love of my blue (gray) pit bull.

SETTING UP YOUR SPACE

Here are some things you can do right now to help make your space feel like a welcoming home! Look at your house like you're a realtor. What is your first impression?

Declutter Your Space

This doesn't necessarily mean you have to live like a minimalist, but rather, have a space for everything and put everything in that space. According to IKEA, 27% of people feel pressure from society to live minimally.[16] There is no one right way to build your home, only what is right for you.

Your bedroom is your place of rest. This is your sanctuary, clear of distractions and clutter. Free of kid toys or laundry, or in my case, dog toys. Turning your bedroom into a warm, sensual, and all-around sexual sanctuary can be achieved in a few simple steps.

Ditch the Technology

"But my phone is my alarm clock!" Yes, I understand, I'm guilty of that too. It's totally fine to have your phone plugged

---

16 "Beyond Four Walls," IKEA Life At Home Report 2018, https://lifeath-ome.ikea.com/wp-content/uploads/2019/09/LAHR18-Report-in-short.pdf.

in next to you, but if there's a power strip next to your side table with enough cables plugged in to it to resemble a snake mating ball, we need to talk. Place the things that are not critically necessary elsewhere, like in the kitchen or office. Again, your bedroom should be your sanctuary, where you can escape the world and create your own.

Upgrade Your Bed

I realize that different styles and designs come with their special touches that make them unique, but try to choose bedding that is less college chic and more adult. Consider purchasing a nice sheet set and creating the *hotel effect* at home. Honestly, do not skimp on good sheets. According to a study done by Slumber Cloud, Americans will spend thirty-six years in bed![17] If that isn't motivation to get quality sheets, I don't know what is.

If you're covered on the sheet aspect, consider investing in a quality mattress. This can provide a more restful sleep and create an exciting playground for you and your partner. If a new mattress is not currently in the budget, a mattress pad is a quick way to upgrade your current bed and give it a new feel. The goal behind this is to make sure that your bed is the most luxurious place in your home. (If you can't part from the faux fur cheetah body pillow, that's okay, too.)

---

17 Kate Mellot, "How To Build a Bedder Relationship with Your Bed," Slumber Cloud, last modified March 21, 2019, https://www.slumbercloud.com/blog/better-relationship-with-your-bed/.

Lighting

I think that the lighting in a bedroom can either make or break the mood. The worst lighting for a bedroom is harsh, direct, overhead lighting. No one is flattered in the beams that are cast directly down upon you. Bedroom lighting should be soft, and bedside reading lights or freestanding lamps can achieve that hotel effect. Another often overlooked point is ease of access. Try to make your lighting as easy to reach as possible. No one wants to have to cross the great expanse of a bedroom and hope they don't smash into the dresser. They still make the clapper, right? Your toes will thank you. Also, if you want to illuminate the room with candles, be mindful of the scents you choose. A strongly scented candle can overpower the space of a bedroom, so consider lightly scented or unscented candles. A safer choice would be flameless LED candles that come with a remote—instant ambiance at the click of a button.

Side Table

These are great to keep what you need close by, like your cell phone—ahem, alarm clock—and a glass of water. Consider using a side table that comes with a drawer. Bedside space is then much more versatile, and you can keep things that you may not be as comfortable displaying out in the open, like sex toys, condoms, or your bite guard case. The idea is to keep what you need near you and easily accessible. Again, we want to avoid dark, toe-stubbing trips across the bedroom in search of items. When the time comes, you want to be prepared.

Mirror

This may seem like a next-level bedroom accessory, but hear me out. I'm not sure if a mirror will add to the quality of your sleep, but I know that it can change the dynamic during erotic encounters (with yourself or a partner). I realize that some may feel that introducing a mirror into a bedroom will make them too self-conscious, but it may be just the thing to spark new erotic heights. If you have a large free-standing mirror, strategically place it so you can catch glimpses of yourself in it. Since you will already have the perfect lighting in your bedroom, as recommended above, you will be set up for sex-cess. When you're ready, you can move it closer or decide that it is better suited facing away from you. You'll never know unless you try.

See your bedroom in a new light. From functional to sensual, a carefully curated and thoughtful bedroom can be easily achieved, and the benefits are nearly endless.

HOW TO GET OUT OF A FUNK

Sometimes, no matter our "before the bad day plan," our healing crystals, and all of our lavender essential oil, we can sometimes find ourselves in a funk. This is absolutely normal. You get to have bad days. Bad days are a great time to practice mindfulness. Mindfulness is the practice of sitting with what is happening right now, without wishing it were different—being present and accepting of the current state of things, both the pleasant and unpleasant. And when the unpleasant feelings come, don't worry, they will not be there forever.

OTHER COMPONENTS OF SELF-CARE

Stress management: Accept what you are in control of and what you aren't. Hopefully, the tips we've previously mentioned will help reduce stressful situations or better prepare you to cope with them.

Nutrition: I will expand more on this in our section on body image, but it deserves a mention here. Are you eating? Are you fueling your body? Don't think that you need to complete a task first in order to deserve food. Eat something and continue on your way.

Sleep and time management: This circles back to protecting that schedule. This means allocating your time and availability to specific things and sticking to it. Have you allocated enough time for what you need to get done? Have you allotted time for rest? I mostly feel strongly about having a dedicated "shut it down" time so you can have rest and leisure without the feeling of guilt that you "should" be doing work instead. It may take a few tries before you can nail down a schedule that works with your daily life.

Be engaged, stay active: Make sure you have time allotted for connections and activities that bring you joy. Much of our waking time is spent working, so make sure that your rest time is factored in as a priority as well.

Talk about boundaries: Sometimes when we're activating our new self-care plan, friends or family may feel slighted that we've decided to choose ourselves over something with them. But it's important to shift our mindset and qualify self-care as a necessity, rather than a luxury. Keep in mind that those who do not respect your boundaries do not respect you.

Massage: The benefits of massage are widely known, and results from massage include reduced anxiety, headaches, and muscle tension; decreased stress-related insomnia; better digestion; and more. This healing power of touch can also evoke feelings of comfort and connection (remember skin hunger?). While there is often a cost associated with this kind of activity, consider treating yourself to one every now and then. You can even benefit from self-massage, and that's free! Again, massage can be part of a luxurious pamper day, but it doesn't mean that massage is an extravagance. It is a powerful tool that you can include in your self-care routine.

Yoga: I cannot sing the praises of yoga enough. This form of exercise is available to all body types and gives you both a mind and body workout. The lessons you learn on the mat can be applied to so many other areas of your life. In addition to gaining flexibility, you gain a greater appreciation for your body. You become more aware of how your body exists in its environment and what you're feeling. Through the various poses, you get an internal massage that can help detoxify your body, as well as a fresh infusion of oxygenated blood.

Research has shown that yoga has the ability to improve balance, increase flexibility, and reduce lower back pain. Bringing awareness to your body through this practice while flowing and breathing though the positions is its own kind of special gift. Consider adding a practice into your lifestyle. It can even be as short as five minutes. Yoga meets you where you are. You don't need anything fancy, just a body and a place to practice.

CHAPTER 3:

SELF-LOVE
MASTURBATION AND FANTASY

A lot of our sexual hang-ups can stem from our upbringing. Messages about sex and masturbation can be pushed on us way before we've even considered the act itself. By examining these teachings from our youth, we can start to unlearn the harmful messages we received and gain back our confidence.

Once we feel empowered to explore the realms of masturbation, fantasy, and sex toys, we can use self-love to discover new paths to pleasure, no partner needed (batteries might be required). We can also teach ourselves more about our own bodies and preferences, which will come in handy when we do have the opportunity to play with other people.

VIRGINITY AS A SOCIAL CONSTRUCT

Virginity is a social construct. That is to say, it is made up by society. There is no medical or scientific definition of virginity. This is just another way we police bodies.

The idea of virginity often finds prevalence in religious beliefs. Virginity is often traditionally seen as something that is valued, particularly in women—and "taking virginity" can mean more gain for someone else, particularly men. But this traditional notion of virginity takes away the bodily autonomy of women. It also adds more pressure around sex, by adding a layer of stigma and shame.

There is no physical manifestation that happens to penis owners when they "lose their virginity"—we are just left to take their word for it. People will often cite the hymen as an indicator of whether or not someone with a vagina has had penetrative sex. This, too, is such an inaccurate belief. The hymen, which is tissue that can partly cover the vaginal opening, comes in all sorts of configurations. The tissue thins as the body reaches puberty and needs to be open for menstrual fluid to escape.

The notion that a hymen will be "broken" and bleed when a person "loses their virginity" is another common misconception, yet some people still believe that. Apparently, some fathers accompany their daughters to gynecological exams and ask the doctor to perform a "virginity" test on them. Holy gross, Batman. In truth, plenty of people no longer have much hymen tissue remaining by the time they have sex. Hymens can also be "broken" by a variety of activities like sports, riding a bike, or inserting a tampon. *IF* there is some remaining tissue that is covering the vaginal opening, it may stretch or tear during penetrative sex, and some blood may be present.

Some people find the idea of virginity so appealing that they will purposely have a "revirgination" surgery in which their hymen is partially reconnected so that the next time they have sex, there is the tearing and bleeding that is traditionally a sign that someone was indeed a virgin.

Placing so much pressure on remaining sex free can have an extremely detrimental effect on someone's sexual life. Someone who has been indoctrinated in the belief that sexuality is bad or dangerous can struggle to find pleasure in future encounters. Also, what do we say to sexual assault victims who perhaps had their first sexual experience against their will? The whole belief system needs to be thrown out. If anything, let's call it a sexual debut and you can decide who and what counts for yourself.

CORN FLAKES AND MICHIGAN

For those who may not know, Michigan is my home state. Despite not being a large state, it is home to many companies based in our pleasant peninsula. In addition to being the automotive capital of the country, we are host to the global headquarters of the Kellogg Company, the producers and inventors of corn flakes. Now, as innocuous as this breakfast cereal may seem, its history is one that is filled with ulterior motives and lucky breaks.

According to the Seventh-day Adventist Church, which incidentally has its origins in Battle Creek as well, a low-fat vegetarian diet is recommended, as per their teachings. Church member John Kellogg was a physician and the superintendent of the Battle Creek Sanitarium. All of the patients there were required to adopt a diet that consisted of mostly bland foods. He believed that consumption of anything spicy or sweet would increase sexual desires, which he was in staunch opposition to.[18] Go abstinence? The thought behind eating bland foods was to curb sexual urges.

---

18 John H. Kellogg, *Plain Facts for Old and Young* (I. F. Segner, 1882), https://www.google.com/books/edition/Plain_Facts_for_Old_and_Young/yyUKAAAAIAAJ?hl=en&gbpv=0.

He and his brother, Will Keith Kellogg, began a whole grain cereal production company in an effort to help promote their belief in bland meals for health. And as the story goes, one day the two accidentally left some cooked wheat out because they had to deal with an issue at the sanitarium. When they came back, they saw that their cooked wheat had turned stale, but they couldn't afford to throw it away. They processed the stale cooked wheat through the grain rollers, and unexpectedly, they got flakes. They then toasted the flakes and began to serve them to their patients. It was an instant hit. John Kellogg later applied for a patent on his "flake process," and corn flakes were born.[19]

So how does this tie into sex? As I mentioned before, Dr. Kellogg was an advocate for sexual abstinence, and being a supporter of Sylvester Graham's agenda (yes, the guy graham crackers are named after) he believed that eating meals of boring, plain old, unsexy corn flakes would help alleviate sufferers from their sexual urges. Specifically, Graham believed that this sort of diet would reduce masturbation, which he believed was detrimental to health. Keep it bland and vegetarian to quell sexual feelings. Luckily, we know the diet didn't work, as many people enjoy corn flakes and graham crackers and still lead sexually fulfilling lives. The only way these work as a detriment to sex is if you eat them in bed and drop crumbs.

---

19   Mary Cross, *A Century of American Icons*, (Greenwood Press, 2002), https://archive.org/details/centuryofamerica00cros/page/12/mode/2up.

HYSTERIA AND THE HISTORY OF MASTURBATION

Often times we've been told that the main event for sex is supposed to be penetrative PV (penis in vagina) sex. But when you find yourself single, penetrative sex can be hard to come by because you're alone. (Not to mention, the idea that "real sex is PV sex" is problematic for innumerable other reasons, including the fact that it erases or delegitimizes the vibrant sex lives of many folks in the LGBTQ+ community.) We need to shift away from that old idea that masturbation is somehow a subpar form of sexuality, left to those who cannot "get" sex elsewhere. A last resort.

It's easy to say just "go masturbate," but sometimes getting around those mental blocks requires unlearning what we have been told by society, family, or other cultural and religious institutions. And these stories are hard to unlearn. Back in the day, masturbation was cited as the culprit for such ailments as acne, insanity, hairy palms, and even premature death. (Despite all of these supposed maladies, I assure you that masturbation is a safe and healthy activity.) Dr. Kellogg had an entire section in his book detailing both the dangers of masturbation and the subsequent "treatments" for the prevention.[20] The proposed methods to keep people from self-polluting ranged from mild to barbaric. Also, chastity devices were used, but those have been around since long before Kellogg encouraged people to lock up the cock.

Starting in the late 1800s up until 1980 (when it was

---

20 John H. Kellogg, *Plain Facts for Old and Young* (I. F. Segner, 1882), https://www.google.com/books/edition/Plain_Facts_for_Old_and_Young/yyUKAAAAIAAJ?hl=en&gbpv=0.

finally removed from the DSM—the Diagnostic and Statistical Manual of Mental Disorders), there was also a condition known as "hysteria" that was said to be plaguing women. Almost any ailment could be covered under the blanket diagnosis of hysteria: things like shortness of breath, fainting (umm hello corsets), depression, anxiety, irritability, you name it! It was believed that a "wandering uterus" was the cause of the problems. So how did one deal with a wandering uterus? Nowadays we'd likely have the Target PA system call out to the misbehaving uterus and tell her to meet us by the customer service desk, but we live in a modern time.

Back then, doctors would perform a massage to provoke a "hysterical paroxysm" in their patients. To read between the lines, the doctor would stimulate the patient until she would have an orgasm. But of course, back then, this was purely medicinal. I'm sure as word spread of this miracle treatment, women were lining up to be treated with this curative measure. Treating the growing number of patients who were suffering from hysteria became an exhausting job for the doctor. Eventually someone had the idea to create a machine to do the hard work for them! Enter: the vibrator. Again, this is not a sex toy . . . yet.

Now, sex toys are nothing new. They have been around for a very, very long time. Originally they were carved from materials such as stone. One of the oldest sex toys on record is a siltstone phallus. It was found in Germany and said to date back twenty-eight thousand years![21] Fast forward to the

---

21 Jonathan Amos, "Ancient Phallus Unearthed in Cave," BBC News, last modified July 25, 2005, http://news.bbc.co.uk/2/hi/science/nature/4713323.stm.

1920s, and popular brands like Hamilton Beach were selling therapeutic "home massagers." These could be found in catalogs, and you could order them and have them sent to your home.

These massagers weren't seen as sex toys, but of course, as time went on, people started to understand their most practical applications. Sexually conservative people realized that "Hey! This is sexual and we don't like that!" and the contraptions were shunned and pushed into the dark, like a dirty thing from the past that we'd like to forget.

Fast forward to the present time—at the writing of this book, the year 2020—and while some cities like New York, Los Angeles, and San Francisco host entire Sex Expos to sell a wide variety of sex toys, it is still illegal to purchase sex toys in some places (lookin' at you, Alabama[22]).

MASTURBATION BENEFITS

Masturbation can be the turning point for a lot of people when it comes to making peace with their bodies. Understanding that you are worthy of sexual pleasure is so powerful. You, in whatever body, right now, can and deserve to experience pleasure.

This is where self-love comes in. During a time when you may not have access to a sexual partner, or to someone who respects you and isn't exploitative, you can be the director of your own sexual satisfaction. By embracing masturbation, not only do you get to learn how to pleasure yourself in a way that you like, you can learn to better communicate the ways

22 Alabama Code Title 13A. Criminal Code § 13A-12-200.2. https://codes. findlaw.com/al/title-13a-criminal-code/al-code-sect-13a-12-200-2.html.

that you like to be touched, if and when you decide to add a partner to the mix.

Your skin can get a boost from masturbation too! And no, it's not going to cause blindness. Immediately following orgasm, people can see what we in the industry like to call the *afterglow.* Typically your skin is flushed post-orgasm due to increased blood flow, and you just look so darn happy! The best kept secret to glowing skin is literally at your fingertips.

Research[23] has shown that people who engage in sexual activity often report less stress in their lives, which can lower the hormone reaction that causes inflammation, one of the many causes of acne and wrinkles. Also, the increased blood flow helps add to that youthful, fresh-faced look.

Research[24] has also shown that orgasms (and the accompanying oxytocin) can help alleviate pain. So the next time menstrual cramps are bringing you down, why not try some natural relief in the form of masturbation?

Adding some self-loving sessions into your life is a great way to not only honor yourself, but to reap these great benefits. Try to find a time when you can fit it in, in a place where you won't be interrupted, and have at it! Mood boosting, stress reducing, skin benefits—and best of all, it's free!

23   Kerstin Uvnas-Moberg et al., "Oxytocin is a Principal Hormone that Exerts Part of its Effects by Active Fragments," *Medical Hypotheses* 133 (December 2019), https://doi.org/https://doi.org/10.1016/j.mehy.2019.109394.

24   Ibid.

SEX TOYS MYTHS

Let's delve in to some of the most prevalent myths about sex toys:

Sex toys are only for lonely people that can't get sex from someone else: We already established that this is untrue. Single people and people in relationships can benefit from the use of a sex toy.

Sex toys are for women only: Very untrue. Sex toys are made for all kinds of bodies. In fact, there are some sex toys for penis owners that give me my own kind of penis envy.

People who use sex toys are lacking in their normal sex life: Sex toys can be part of a person's normal sex life. Someone's sex life can look very different from yours, and that doesn't make it wrong or somehow less normal.

Sex toys are expensive: While your hands are free, sex toys generally do cost money. You don't have to break the bank, though, when it comes to purchasing a toy (more on that in the following sections).

My partner will think I'm a freak if I ask to introduce a toy into bed: Absolutely. Kidding! There may be some hesitancy from a partner who isn't familiar with sex toys or who believes that it is a slight against them and their sexual prowess, but help them understand that a sex toy can work as a complementary part of your sex life. You aren't replacing them with the toy, just adding it to make things even hotter.

TYPES OF SEX TOYS

Fear not! Sex toys have come a long way since their stone-carved ancestors. When it comes to pleasure, there are so many options to use. Here are a few common toys.

Dildo

This is a nonvibrating object that can be inserted into your vagina or anus. Dildos can be straight or have a curve, often resembling a penis. The length and girth can vary. And if we're going to be putting it in our butt, it must have a flared base. Dildos can mimic the feel of PV sex and provide greater penetration than your fingers alone. It can also stimulate areas like the G-spot, which can sometimes be challenging to reach.

Fun Fact An easy phrase to remember when it comes to anything anal is "without a base, without a trace." Meaning, if whatever you inserted into your butt does not have a flared base or isn't attached to a human body, it's likely going to get lost. This then requires a trip to the emergency room and a lot of questions.

In 2019, the US Consumer Product Safety Commission[25] released their annual list of things people put in their butts:

- Dildo
- Vibrator
- Prostate toy

---

25 United States Consumer Product Safety Commission, "NEISS Highlights, Data and Query Builder," last modified 2019, https://www.cpsc.gov/cgibin/NEISSQuery/home.aspx.

▸ String

▸ A pencil

▸ Bouncy ball

▸ Some marbles

▸ Crayon

▸ Aerosol can

▸ Pen

▸ Ear buds

▸ Balloon full of heroin

▸ Anal beads

▸ Small bottle of baby oil

▸ Bottle

▸ Bag of molly

Vibrator

This is essentially any toy that has vibrational capabilities. Vibrators can come in many different shapes and be used in a variety of locations. Far from the steam-powered vibrators from our hysteria history, nowadays vibrators can be as small and discreet as a tube of lipstick. A vibrator is one of the most commonly used sex toys. As most women require clitoral stimulation to reach orgasm, a vibrator is the perfect tool for the job. A vibrator can also be used during penetration (say, from your dildo) to help you reach orgasm as well. Some sex toys include a dual motor, with a vibrating insertable part and a vibrating clitoral part. And in order to be considered a rabbit-style vibrator, the insertable part has to have some moving component. Whether that is a thrusting motion or rotating beads, it has to move.

Butt Plug

This toy is designed to plug up your butt, as the name implies. These toys can create a feeling of fullness that some people find sexually arousing.

Any time we're talking about butt stuff, a conversation about lube is sure to happen. Additional lubricant is required whenever we're doing any kind of anal play. The anus does not naturally lubricate; therefore, we need to bring some to the party (more on lube later). This toy is meant to stay inside of you while you go about stimulating yourself in other ways. If the thought of anal play with repeated entry and exit excites you, consider anal beads.

Anal Beads

This toy is designed to be inserted and removed from your butt. Often made of graduated beads, which start small and gradually size up, anal beads can be used to stimulate your anus by playing with your sphincter. Look for a toy that is made of one continuous material. There are some that are on a rope (I don't know why they're still making them), but that can never be properly cleaned, so stick with something that can be cleaned post use. Many cite the onset of climax as the best time to remove anal beads. It can provide a unique sensation and add to the contractions of your orgasm.

Nipple Clamps

Many women report experiencing pleasurable feelings from nipple stimulation. Nipple clamps can be a soft sensation or a serious pinch. Experiment with different sensations and find a setting that gives you your favorite kind of touch.

BUYING SEX TOYS

Shopping for a vibrator these days couldn't be easier! The internet holds an endless amount of options for you. There are many adult shops all over the country (unless you are in Alabama), and now you can even find vibrators in mainstream grocery stores. Whether you're looking to buy your first vibrator or you're a seasoned professional, here are some things to consider when shopping for your latest sex accessory.

Size and Power

Are you looking for something that is compact and discreet, or are you looking for something with all of the bells and whistles? Do you want one that is phallic shaped or something more contemporary? Just like snowflakes, vibrators come in all shapes and sizes. Also, size is not directly correlated with vibration power. If you can, test out the vibration strength and see if it's right for you before you buy it.

Sexologist tip for those with vaginas: try the vibe on the tip of your nose to really get an idea of how it will feel on your clitoris. You have a similar amount of nerve endings on the tip of your nose as you do on your clitoris. Maybe that's why they say a sneeze is an eighth of an orgasm?

Energy

How does your toy get its buzz? There are many power options for vibrators these days. Some are powered by batteries. Some are rechargeable. Some need to be plugged in, and there are even ones that are solar powered! Find out which one is right for you. With a corded vibrator, there is no doubt that you will have power, but it may limit your options due to the cord length. Those that are powered by batteries or rechargeable are more mobile, but if you let the battery die down, you may literally have created your own buzzkill.

Noise

Does it sound like you are making a smoothie, or is it whisper soft? Are the neighbors going to complain? Different vibrators have different levels of loudness. Again, turn it on and try it out if you can. If sound doesn't matter to you, the sky's the limit! If you have roommates, children, or nosy neighbors, maybe a quieter vibe is for you. Decide what level is right for you so that you don't get distracted from the task at hand.

Material

What is the vibrator made of? There are lots of sex toys on the market that are made from low-quality rubbers and plastics. Read the box and look for toys that are phthalate free. Phthalates are used in soft plastics and are associated with health risks. Do you want a more realistic, skin-like vibrator, a funky textured feel, or a smooth, sleek surface? Different materials come with different types of smells, and keep in mind that different materials require different cleaning techniques, too. Also, will your toy need to be latex compatible? What about lubricants? Try to be mindful of all of these considerations as you shop around.

Price

How much are you hoping to spend on your sex accessory? There are price points ranging from a few dollars to a few million. The Pearl Royale is one of the most expensive sex toys in the world. Valued at 1.3 million dollars, it is made of platinum and studded with precious gems and pearls. Keep in mind that price isn't necessarily an indication of the vibrator's quality. Weigh your options on what you want in a toy, and see where that lands you on the price continuum. You can find many quality sex toys that will fit your budget and won't lack on power.

FANTASY

When we're talking about masturbation, we often have to talk about fantasy. Fantasy is a powerful tool in creating sexual feelings and arousal. Sometimes visual images are not enough to sexually arouse us, so we have to use our brains. The human brain is one of our most powerful sexual organs. When we think of fantasy, literally the sky's the limit! Or, like in *Mean Girls*, "The limit does not exist."

Since the brain is one of our largest sexual organs, it's no surprise that fantasy plays such an important role in our satisfaction. I want to first dispel any myths around the idea that we should not be fantasizing about other people, situations, or even taboo things, whether single or not. This is complete nonsense. Fantasy has been a pillar of our existence since we were born. Clearly the turn toward sexual fantasy happened as we aged, but nonetheless, it's here to stay and completely normal.

Some people feel that fantasizing about anything but their partner may constitute some kind of cheating, but that isn't true. Oftentimes fantasy is the thing we need to reach our sexual satisfaction. Try masturbating while assembling an ingredient list for taco night. It's hard to complete either task. Fantasy is our chance to enhance what we may be experiencing physically and explore the unknown, safely within the constraints of our mind.

Many people report a fantasy about being sexually taken by force. Does this mean that people are seeking out rape encounters? No. Rather, they might be drawn to the aggression, the shift in power, and the ferocity of it. Perhaps they are drawn to the loss of control, the feeling of helplessness or submission, or even to the fact that it's taboo. This is just a fantasy, though, and imagining something does not necessarily mean that you want it to happen in real life.

It's also important to note that sometimes our fantasies are better left in the land of make believe, rather than trying to experience them in reality. Fantasies like group sex, threesomes, or passionate sex make their way to the top of the list for some. Fantasies can also be a beacon for what we're seeking out in our sexual lives. For instance, someone who fantasizes about very passionate, slow sex, may be craving that kind of encounter IRL. Am I dreaming about painting my fantasy lover's chest in Nutella and licking it off while taking breaks to kiss them with my sweet, chocolatey lips right now? One big licking YES. Do I want to do that in real life? Probably not. Chocolate stains sheets and, knowing me, those sugar-covered lips would end up on my vulva and I'd be welcoming a yeast infection. Sometimes fantasies can just stay fantasies.

If we frame our qualification of a good sexual encounter to mean that everyone is sexually satisfied and content, this opens up the door to many more opportunities for a good sexual encounter to occur. More specifically, if we can achieve sexual satisfaction with ourselves, we don't have to worry about looking for it in others. Maybe you had amazing mind-blowing sex with a partner, and now you're worried that you're single and this might not be available to you ever again. I challenge you to be your own best lover.

Once we have become our own best lovers, we will be better able to articulate our likes and dislikes to future partners. Also, as your sexual satisfaction grows within yourself, a side effect of that is commonly an increase in body confidence (more on that later). The better you feel about the skin you live in, the more comfortable and confident you will be in the world.

Journal prompt: To better help you exercise your creative juices, try to write down things you can feel, but not easily see. This can help you during times when you're calling on fantasy while masturbating.

KEGELS

Many of you may be familiar with the term *Kegel*, but do you know the history? The exercise and term were coined by gynecologist Arnold Kegel in the late '40s. He was the creator of the Kegel perineometer, which measured the strength of voluntary contractions of the pelvic floor, and the subsequent Kegel exercises. Described as a repeated contraction and relaxation of the pelvic floor muscles, Kegel exercises are important and beneficial to many.

Contrary to popular belief, people at all stages of life can benefit from exercising their pelvic floor. Doing Kegel exercises strengthens the pelvic floor muscles for stronger contractions during orgasm, and helps with a condition called urinary incontinence. Women who are post-baby, menopausal, or overweight can experience involuntary leakage of urine.[26] The most common types of urinary incontinence are stress urinary (usually due to pelvic damage from childbirth) or urge urinary incontinence (abnormal bladder contractions). A laugh, a sneeze, a cough, or the lifting of weight can bring on an unwanted leak and really put a damper on things (pun intended).

If you are in the category above and currently living with urinary incontinence, you're in luck! Pelvic floor muscle training (PFMT) is often one of the first things a medical professional will prescribe to combat urinary incontinence. The human body is an amazing marvel, and with simple exercise, muscles that are damaged or weak can heal. A study published in *BJOG: An International Journal of Obstetrics and Gynaecology* found that women benefited from PFMT during late pregnancy to prevent and treat urinary incontinence.[27] Another study published in the *Handbook of Sports Medicine and Science: The Female Athlete* found that training of the pelvic floor muscles led to an increase in muscle thickness and lift, which can assist in treating pelvic organ prolapse.[28]

This is all well and good, but how do you do the Kegel

---

26 Leslee L. Subak et al,. "Obesity and Urinary Incontinence: Epidemiology and Clinical Research Update," *The Journal of Urology* 182, no. 6 (December 2009), https://doi.org/10.1016/j.juro.2009.08.071.

27 E.T.C. Reilly et al., "Prevention of Postpartum Stress Incontinence in Primigravidae with Increased Bladder Neck Mobility: A Randomised Controlled Trial of Antenatal Pelvic Floor Exercises," *BJOG: An International Journal of Obstetrics and Gynaecology* 109, no. 1: 68–76, https://www.sciencedirect.com/science/article/abs/pii/S1470032802011163.

28 Margot L. Mountjoy, *Handbook of Sports Medicine and Science: The Female Athlete* (Wiley-Blackwell, 2014), https://onlinelibrary.wiley.com/doi/10.1002/9781118862254.ch8.

exercises? The greatest thing about Kegels is that you can do them anywhere. While brushing your teeth, at stoplights, in the elevator, waiting in line at the grocery store—the locations are endless! I'm doing them right now as I type this.

For those of you who may be unfamiliar with which muscle groups we are trying to target, the easiest way to locate them is the stop/start technique. The next time you are urinating, try to stop and start the flow of urine. Ta-da! You've found the muscles! Now that you've found the muscles, it's time to exercise. I do not recommend using the stop/start method of urination to exercise; use it only as a guide to finding your muscles. Continuing to use the stop/start method as exercise can lead to incomplete emptying of the bladder.

The simplest way to start a Kegel regimen is to lift and hold your muscles for five seconds and relax your muscles for five seconds. Try to repeat this five times in one sitting. You can work your way up to holding and relaxing for ten seconds at a time. Once you've mastered this entry-level exercise, you can gradually increase time. It is important to note that the exercising of the pelvic floor muscles is not the act of bearing down. This can actually loosen the muscles and disrupt all of your hard work.

Now that you're doing Kegels, how do you know if you're making progress? Your pelvic floor may become sore, gain tolerance, and with regular exercising, increase in strength. Eventually, the hope is that it will alleviate issues such as accidental leakage.

As with any exercise, you will not see huge gains in the first days, but over time, you should notice a marked difference from where you were before starting your exercise routine. Considering one in three women will experience urinary incontinence in their life, talking about this problem and having actionable solutions is imperative to all of us.

LUBE

When we are aroused, our bodies often respond by producing lubrication. This can be a lot, a little, or even none at all. The amount of lubrication is not reflective of how aroused you are. There are many factors like health, hydration, and hormones that can impact the ability to produce natural lubrication.

The lubrication produced in the vagina helps facilitate penetration by reducing friction between the vagina and whatever is being inserted into it. But we don't only have PV sex, and most of us are not having sex just to procreate. We engage in all kinds of sexual activities and sometimes our natural lubrication can't keep up with the duration of our sex sessions. The use of lube is NOT a sign that you aren't turned on enough, and it's not a cop-out. Lube is a great staple to include in your solo and partnered sex life.

Lube comes in many different varieties. Lubes can be water, silicone, or oil based, and each of these has their benefits. Some things to keep in mind while lube shopping:

Water Based

Water-based lubricant is, as the name implies, based off of water. This lube is safe for use with condoms and toys. It is easily washed away and won't stain your sheets. The only drawback to this kind of lubricant is that it isn't very long lasting. People often complain of sticky lube because they were using water-based lubricant, it dried out, and then they added more lube. What you need to do is add more water to reactivate the lubricant. Water-based lubricants are also very inexpensive.

Flavored lubes are usually water based and are great for oral sex. Although, I would caution you to try them before you buy them, if you can. You don't want it to taste like cough medicine—unless that's your thing. You can usually find small sample sized packs of lube, flavored and regular, in stores. Think of it like bulk candy: buy a bunch and see which ones you like! Also exercise caution whenever using flavored lubricants around the vagina. Depending on the sweetener, your vagina may have an adverse reaction to it. Every body is different, so testing on yourself is key.

Silicone Based

Silicone lube is great for extended play and anal play because it won't dry out as quickly as water-based lubricant, but the taste can be unpleasant, and clean-up can be a little more involved. It is latex friendly, but be mindful if you're going to use it with a toy that's made of a silicone composite. The two together will cause your toy to disintegrate and become sticky, and no one likes a sticky dildo.

Hybrid Based

This is the best of both worlds. You get the longevity of the silicone lube and the slippery quality from a water-based lubricant. (Hybrid-based lubricants might affect some silicone toys, but it depends on the chemical composition of the toy. Best practice is to do a spot test on your toy to see what happens before using them together in a sexual scenario.)

Oil Based

Many people are into oil-based lubricants as well. These are fine to use on yourself, but not great if you plan on using a latex condom with it. The oil can degrade the latex and cause it to break. Coconut oil is a good option to use during sex since it closely resembles the oil naturally produced on skin and can be organic. Coconut oil also has some antibacterial and antifungal properties that can be appealing to some. Important note: if you choose to use an oil-based lubricant, be sure to check that nothing is added to the oil product, since added sugars or other ingredients might lead to issues like yeast infections. Plain, virgin, organic oils only!

Anal Lubricant

Some lubes are touted as "anal specific" because they contain the numbing chemical benzocaine, but I caution your use of these. Pain is your body's way of indicating something is wrong. You need to know when something is hurting, and being numb in the rear region can inadvertently lead to injuries.

HOW TO MASTURBATE

Basically, there are no rules. Whatever gives your body pleasure! Some folks enjoy touching, stroking, rubbing, tapping, grinding, vibrating, suctioning, and otherwise playing with their genitals. But pay attention to the rest of your body, too. So many hot spots beyond your genitals can be pleasured. In fact, I encourage you to discover new areas of excitement before going to your known hotspots.

Set the scene. Make a nest. Immerse yourself in the most comfortable environment that you can. Maybe that means adding some extra blankets and pillows to your bed, turning off the lights, and lighting a few candles—or maybe even killing the lights altogether and letting your hands and imagination explore in the dark. Swipe on that airplane mode! Once you've created your ideal environment, think of something hot. Something that sexually arouses you. If you're having difficulty coming up with a scenario in your head, look to media for inspiration. Is there a book passage that you find particularly hot? Maybe you want to watch some porn to stoke the fire? Whatever you need to do is perfectly okay!

Once you're comfortable, start touching your body. You can absolutely go for your hottest spots first, but I challenge you to take your time. Slow it down and caress yourself all over. Feel what it's like to touch yourself in a way that pleases you.

Once you've built up enough anticipation, it's time to switch gears. Go ahead and touch your hottest spots. If you have a sex toy, now might be the time to tag it into the party. Lubricant is always great to have on hand to help reduce friction for a slippery good time.

Being partnerless doesn't mean that you're removed from receiving sexual pleasure. This is a time when you can explore sex on your own, unhurried, and potentially nonstop. Give yourself permission to fully explore all of your body, and to relish in all of the pleasure you can bring yourself!

CHANGE UP YOUR MASTURBATION HABIT

There is some definite truth in the saying "If it ain't broke, don't fix it." It makes sense not to change something that is already working well for you. But as curious creatures, we can most definitely be open to trying new things. Sometimes simply changing the positioning of your body can be an exciting new twist to your self-love game.

If you frequently masturbate on your back in bed, try it on your stomach. This gives you a different tactile sensation on your breasts and belly. Also, you can try grinding on a pillow. If you'd like to completely skip the bed, think about the bathroom. Cue the waterworks. But instead of tears, think faucets.

If you have a bathtub with faucet access, position your body under the flow of water. Check the temperature first! Make sure it's pleasant, so you aren't freezing or scalding your vulva. What's great with water is that you can adjust the flow of water to be a gentle trickle over your clitoris or your own personal Niagara Falls. Don't despair if you only have access to a showerhead. If it's fixed on, you can inexpensively purchase a removable showerhead and swap them out. Find a setting that you enjoy and stimulate yourself with the shower head.

Try to masturbate with a toy or by humping something. People have been getting off for thousands of years, so it's safe to say that there are infinite ways to bring about your pleasure.

CHAPTER 4:
BODY MAPPING

Body mapping is a way for you to have a full users'
guide, if you will, of how your body works and feels,
and what it enjoys. I'm sure you can list off the ways your
body is feeling right now, but how would you respond if I
asked you how your lower back feels when fingertips are on
it? Be real with me here, did you just put your fingertips
on your back to see what that felt like? Keep that curiosity
going with the rest of your body.

Writing down or saying how our body feels in response to
different stimuli can be helpful when recalling what kind of
touch is most appreciated where. Feel free to do a body scan
any time something in life has impacted you, like an injury,
illness, or childbirth. These things could have changed the
way you feel about certain areas being touched.

SENSATE FOCUS

In the 1960s Dr. William Masters and Virginia Johnson, sex
researcher pioneers, developed a sex therapy technique they
called Sensate Focus. The goal of this exercise is to help you

focus on sensory perception (how does this really feel?) and sensuality. Like a crock pot, low and slow is the way to go. This exercise is also not orgasm focused. As much of sexuality is trying to race toward the "goal" (orgasm), this technique takes away the pressure and actually says, "don't."

Despite being over sixty years old, this practice is still used and just as effective today. It has been used to treat things like body image, erectile dysfunction, orgasm disorders, and lack of sexual arousal. Sensate focus is a tool that you can turn to again and again. The more you touch your skin and get to know your body, the greater an understanding you will have about your likes and dislikes. Revel in all of the sensations your body can produce, and notice how and when it comes alive.

Though finding a partner isn't necessarily your goal, this practice also translates into a valuable benefit when/if you find yourself with a new partner because you'll know exactly what feels best and what they should steer clear of.

HOW TO DO SENSATE FOCUS

Carve out twenty-five minutes of your day and situate yourself in a comfortable area where you aren't likely to be disturbed. Surround yourself with comfortable things like cozy pillows or pleasant aromas. We're trying to set a soft and sensual mood, so avoid the blinding lights of a surgery suite.

Set your timer and begin touching your body. Try different strokes, types of touches, and levels of pressure, and note the differences. Does one kind of touch feel better than another?

Nongenital touching: This initial step in sensate focus is for drawing out sensation. You can start anywhere that you like, just make sure you're exploring all of yourself (except your genitals—we are avoiding the genitals right now). What sensations are you able to feel? Does a specific kind of touch feel better or worse? Try out different touches like massaging the area, applying firm pressure, or feather-soft pressure. What about some percussive taps? Flicking? Circles? Do nails feel good against that area? There is no destination with this, just the experience.

Genital touching: As in the previous step, follow the same technique, but this time, touching your genitals. Try to see by using your fingertips. Again, no rush. The idea here is to be present while experiencing all of the sensations you're creating. Also, feel free to add lubricant.

Add lotion: While caressing your skin feels nice, adding a lotion or oil can change the way you perceive your flesh and the way your touch feels. Be mindful if you're using a lotion or oil around the genitals. While it's okay to use them on external skin, getting any kind of lotion or oil in the vagina or urethra can be troublesome and lead to unwanted irritation or infections.

BODY MAPPING: EXPANDING SENSATE FOCUS

This is a verbal exercise. The next time you do the sensate focus with yourself, I want you to verbalize all the sensations that you're feeling in your body. I want it to be a clear depiction of what's going on with you. Again, find a place of comfort in the nest you built, and be present (focused on the present moment). Tap into mindfulness and observe what's happening around you without wishing things were different. What sensations are arising in your body? Tell me how the weight of your body is pressing into the mattress. What is your body saying to you? If your body is telling you an area is painful or sore to the touch, take stock of that. Try to put words to all of your senses. Your fingertips may feel cold on your skin. Your breasts may feel like a warm pink turning red when you massage them. You might feel wetness building between your legs.

This exercise may take a few times to get used to. It can seem weird to verbalize these kinds of sensations, but the more we start to give voice to the feelings that our body parts are experiencing, and pay attention to what they're telling us, the more we will be able to create a map of our body.

EROGENOUS ZONES

Erogenous zones are defined as areas that have high concentrations of nerve endings that, when stimulated, can create a sexual response. Now these can be anywhere on a body, but here are a few common ones and maybe some overlooked ones. Feel free to explore these during your sensate focus times.

The Clitoris

If this were *Family Feud* and we polled one hundred people on the number one erogenous zone for women (and other vulva owners), I'm sure an overwhelming majority would say the clitoris. The clitoris is home to over eight thousand nerve endings and is cited as the most common avenue of stimulation for women to reach orgasm. There is more than what meets the eye to the clitoris as well. The entire clitoral complex is quite large, and mostly internal. It includes a head (the external "button" that you can see under the clitoral hood), an internal shaft, and internal legs that extend to either side of the vagina. Much like an iceberg, you cannot see the size of the clitoris from the surface alone. This structure is homologous with a penis, so it too swells with blood and can become erect during sexual arousal.

The Vagina

Often (mistakenly) used when referring to the vulva, the vagina is the opening. This is a soft, fleshy canal in which lubrication is produced. The first third of the vagina is most sensitive to penetration and vibration, while the rest of it responds more to pressure. As sexual arousal builds, the vagina lengthens and undergoes a process called *tenting*, in which the vagina expands and creates space to facilitate easier penetration.

The Penis

With the penis, we have a couple of hotspots to highlight. The glans, or head, of the penis is very sensitive, made from the same homologous tissue as the clitoris. On the underside of the head, connecting it to the shaft, is the frenulum. It's a highly innervated area and very responsive to touch.

The Testicles

These soft parts are temperature and touch sensitive, so be gentle. Notice a line bisecting the flesh vertically? That's the raphe line, and it would love it if you stroked it there.

The Prostate

This is a small, golf ball–sized gland that is responsible for creating the majority of the fluid we see in ejaculate. It is also highly sensitive to direct and indirect touch. Stimulation is said to create very powerful orgasms.

The Perineum

This is the sensitive stretch of skin between the anus and the vulva or testicles. Stimulating it with a firm press of the knuckles can indirectly stimulate the prostate in men.

The Mouth/Lips

Lips hold a high concentration of nerve endings. Lick your lips right now. How did that feel? Could you feel your tongue lave across them? How are they at detecting temperature changes? Next time you take a sip of a warm drink, I want you to think about this page. Also, good hydration keeps lips soft and full, so drink up!

Nipples

Nipples are very sensitive areas. They can respond to temperature changes and can light up nerve endings in the genitals. Both the clitoris and nipples light up similar sections in the brain when stimulated. Some nursing mothers report feeling vaginal contractions while breastfeeding. Nipple stimulation releases oxytocin, the feel good, bonding hormone, which is also released during orgasm. Aren't bodies fascinating!

Ears

Ears are quite the sensitive area. This brings me flashbacks of getting my ears pierced as a child. Some people enjoy having their ears lightly stroked, nibbled, or even sucked on. Also, let's not discount the aural opportunities here. Hearing sounds of sweet nothings or naughty whispers can also fuel the flames of arousal.

The Head

Think about when you're getting your hair washed and how good that feels. The scalp isn't something we usually see on an erogenous zone list, but it's a good one. There are so many nerve endings in the skin, so give it a scratch or a message. A slow head massage on the couch can be just the thing to relax yourself after a long day, or a sudsy wash massage in the shower can heat things up.

The Inner Wrist

The inner wrist is a hotbed of sensation! Look at your wrist right now—chances are you can see your circulatory system at work through the skin. That thin skin is ripe for kissing and licking. It's an overlooked erogenous zone, but won't be after you try it. You can, of course, lick yourself, but this one may be better if done to others.

The Midsection

This area can include the back, side, and stomach region. Using a light touch—like with the tips of your fingers or even a tickler made of feathers—is a great way to activate this skin. Long strokes can create a sensation that will run up and down the body. Don't be surprised if you raise some goose-flesh. Our skin is our largest sexual organ so take advantage of that real estate.

Basically, this is all about touching areas that don't frequently get as much love as the more popularized ones. When we start to receive stimulation in areas that are not often touched, those sensations can feel heightened and can create a more exciting awareness. And these are just suggestions! Erogenous zones are different for different people. Don't feel limited to this list. Explore your body alone to see if you can identify some new ones.

CHAPTER 5:
ORGASM BASICS

Orgasms are often touted as the highlight of a sexual experience, but are they really? An orgasm is classified as a release of muscle tension through a series of muscular contractions and a pleasurable feeling.

Studies have shown that an orgasm can increase the pain threshold to varying degrees.[29] The body is also flooded with endorphins and oxytocin, which can help contribute to feeling better overall.

TYPES OF ORGASM

Just like snowflakes, orgasms can come in many different varieties.

Clitoral

These types of orgasms are had by stimulating the one part of

---

29 Kerstin Uvnas-Moberg and Maria Petersson, "Oxytocin, a Mediator of Anti-Stress, Well-Being, Social Interaction, Growth and Healing," *Zeitschrift fur Psychosomatische Medizin und Psychotherapie* 51, no. 1 (2005): 57–80, https://doi.org/10.13109/zptm.2005.51.1.57.

your body that is purely designated for pleasure: the clitoris! External or internal stimulation can send you over the edge, and those internal structures of the clitoris can help contribute to the next kind of orgasm.

Vaginal/Cervical

These kinds of orgasm happen via penetration. Sigmund Freud famously called these the mature kind of orgasm,[30] despite the fact that only around 25% of women[31] are consistently able to experience them from penetration alone. Interesting to note, though, is that the legs of the clitoris surround the vaginal opening. It is thought that these vaginal orgasms could be a result of internal clitoral stimulation.

G-Spot

A G-spot (more like G-area, as it's a larger map of vaginal real estate rather than one distinguishable landmark) orgasm can occur from just G-spot stimulation alone. This area can be felt through the anterior wall of the vagina. As arousal builds, the texture of the surrounding tissue becomes engorged and it can be easier to feel. Incidentally, stimulating this area on some women can cause them to have the feeling that they need to urinate.

---

30 Kim Wallen and Elisabeth A. Lloyd, "Female Sexual Arousal: Genital Anatomy and Orgasm in Intercourse," *Hormones and Behavior* 59, no. 5 (December 30, 2010): 780–792, https://doi.org/10.1016/j.yhbeh.2010.12.004.

31 Michael Castleman, "The Most Important Sexual Statistic," *Psychology Today* (March 16, 2009), https://www.psychologytoday.com/us/blog/all-about-sex/200903/the-most-important-sexual-statistic.

Anal

Anal orgasms happen through stimulation of the anus. You can also indirectly stimulate the G-spot or prostate through anal play.

Nipple

It is a small percentage, but some people are able to orgasm from nipple stimulation alone. As mentioned in the last chapter, research suggests that when nipples are stimulated, they light up the same sensory pathways as when the genitals are stimulated: the genital sensory cortex. Also, many women report contractions in their genital region during nipple stimulation. This is also reported to happen during breastfeeding.

Combination/Blended

These kinds of orgasms happen when you combine any of the above kinds of stimulations together into an orgasmic symphony.

Wet Dreams

People of any gender can have these. Your body can experience all sorts of changes while you're asleep, so if you've woken up wet and/or aroused, there is a chance you had a wet dream.

EDGING

Cruise Ship Anecdote

I had the honor of being invited on an adults-only "Lifestyle" cruise in 2020. We set sail from Tampa, Florida and headed to the Caribbean. I was telling everyone that this was a clothing optional, adults only cruise! I later realized that it was just topless optional and not the clothing optional scene that I had previously believed. Very glad I noted that distinction before I just whipped off my dress post dinner.

I was brought on to serve as the onboard sexual edutainment. I was going to teach hands on sex classes. That is, everyone's hands on themselves or their partner. My hands were on my slide clicker, I swear.

One of my classes was on edging. Edging is the practice of bringing yourself to the brink of orgasm and then backing away, then repeating the buildup of sensation, and backing off again. As you do this, your sexual arousal will reach new heights, and when you finally reach climax, it should be an explosive one.

After we went over some basic anatomy and techniques, it was time for my participants to put into practice what we had learned. Now, I should specify that within the red room, clothing was indeed optional, and you could engage in sexual acts. As couples began their edging journey, I discreetly stepped behind a screen to allow the guests their privacy. I kept an eye on them and encouraged them as different steps were implemented.

At about the middle of the session, a cute little old lady came up to me. She mentioned that her husband had a penis implant. First of all, I was thrilled that we'd learned about various kinds of penis implants in grad school, and secondly, I was so happy she said something. We talked about the challenges that can arise from having a penis implant, like being only fully soft or fully hard—there is no in-between arousal build-up. She also confessed to me that her partner had never ejaculated with her! I found that fascinating! I asked if he was able to ejaculate when he is masturbating alone, and she said yes, which led me to believe that this wasn't a mechanical issue. I said to try some of the techniques we went over and see how that goes.

The end of the session was nearing, and I had two couples left in the room still practicing their edging. One was the older woman and her partner and the other was a younger couple. I could tell something was happening with my older couple because the sounds her partner was making started to come faster and faster. He was moaning so loudly, and suddenly, he came! Right in his partner's mouth! Cue me dancing quietly like a weirdo behind the screen. I heard them laughing and exclaiming about what had just happened.

They both walked up to me with the biggest smiles, gave me a hug, and told me how amazing it was for both of them. The wife exclaimed, "If I knew all it would take was attending a sex class to have him ejaculate with me, I would have suggested that we attend one sooner."

This, my friends, is how I know I am doing the Lord's work.

How to Edge

Edging isn't just for people in relationships! You can do it too. Incorporate it into your next masturbation session and whenever you have a new partner. Here's how to do it:

Masturbate as you usually do. As you feel your arousal building, walk yourself right up to the edge of orgasm and then stop your stimulation. Let your body calm back down. Begin stimulation again, go to the edge, and back off. As you explore this practice, you'll be able to see how close you can get to the edge without going over. Of course, if you "mess up," the consequence is an orgasm, so it's really a win-win.

When it comes to edging with a partner, you really need to have great communication and observation skills. You'll have to rely on the body cues from your partner and their ability to tell you when they're close. It's a great way to play and explore with each other, and of course, to get to know each other's bodies.

ORGASM GAP

According to a study published in the *Journal of Sexual Medicine*, which studied single men and women of different sexual orientations in the U.S., men (both heterosexual and homosexual) experienced orgasms on average about 85% of the time. In comparison, heterosexual women orgasmed on average about 62% of the time (lesbian women fared much better, orgasming on average 75% of the time).[32] The orgasm gap is real. While it isn't necessary for orgasm to be present at every sexual interaction to define it as a good one, it's still nice when we have them. Talk to your partner about your own experience. If you can have sex, you can talk about orgasms.

---

32 Justin R. Garcia et al., "Variation in Orgasm Occurrence by Sexual Orientation in a Sample of U.S. Singles," *The Journal of Sexual Medicine* 11, no. 11 (November 1, 2014): 2645–2652, https://doi.org/10.1111/jsm.12669.

It may just be as simple as allowing more time for your body to warm up to the sexual arousal.

Just don't start faking your orgasms.

WHY NOT TO FAKE ORGASM

Why would anyone want to fake an orgasm? Are you trying to win an Academy Award from the bedroom? Doubtful. Some do it to get out of a bad sex session, some think that it will please their partner, some don't want to hurt their partner's feelings, and some just want the sexual experience to end more quickly. You may think that it's no big deal and that there isn't any harm in faking it, but by perpetuating the lie, you are doing more harm than good. So if you've ever faked an orgasm, I'm here to tell you to stop it!

When you fake an orgasm, you're telling your partner that what they're doing to you feels great. Odds are that they will remember what you "liked" the last time and pull that out of their bag of tricks the next time you decide to get down. If you don't like the kind of magic they're wielding, you need to stop reinforcing them with your fake orgasms.

Likewise, do you have a tried and true tested move that you use on all of your sexual partners? Before you pat yourself on the back for the puddle-like state that you always leave your partners in, consider that it may have sometimes been a performance. Everyone is not alike. What works for one person may not necessarily be the same for someone else. I imagine many of you are thinking "no one has ever faked an orgasm with me," but I warn you to tread cautiously.

Aside from the porn-worthy moaning, what other cues let you know that your partner experienced an orgasm? Did their pupils dilate? Was a sex flush present? Did their nipples become erect? Was their pulse elevated? Could you feel their involuntary muscle contractions? Were they out of breath? Just some things to consider next time you think you've left your partner in ecstasy.

For those faking orgasms, I imagine many of you are not faking them out of malice—and stroking your partner's ego is always a plus. But there are a lot of downsides to being inauthentic in the bedroom. I'm not saying that you need to confess your fakes in the past, but consider talking to your partner about what you really like. Communication is the key to a better sex life. Speak up when things aren't feeling the way you'd like. Better yet, show them where and how you like to be touched.

There are a lot of reasons why you might be slow to orgasm, or even unable to orgasm. Maybe you've had a lot to drink, or you're riding that plateau but just can't get over the edge. Just let your partner know where you're at. And where is the rule that says you must have an orgasm or else the job isn't done? You don't have to have an orgasm every time—it's perfectly okay not to.

No one wins when one person is staring up at the ceiling waiting for their partner to be done and the other is so desperately trying to please them. Check in with your partner, be communicative, and above all, have fun. Sex is not supposed to be work, so stop with the acting and start with the enjoying.

WHY CAN'T I ORGASM?

As we've noted, around 75% of women do not orgasm from PV sex alone,[33] but what about the women who experience no orgasm at all? Current statistics have that number at around 5–10%. This number seems a bit high to me, but it's very difficult to get funding for studies involving female sexuality. I think there also lies a discrepancy in self-reporting, as some participants may not know if they've had an orgasm or not. I mean, what even is an orgasm?

Because mainstream media often portrays female sexual satisfaction as a woman yelling and thrashing while deep in the throes of ecstasy, it can be difficult to know if we had an orgasm when our own experiences may not reflect that reaction. That isn't to say that you can't have orgasms like that, but it isn't the only way to experience orgasm. You may have one day where you want to scream at the top of your lungs because it feels so good, and another day it may feel like a little pleasurable blip on your radar. Orgasms come in all shapes and sizes and intensities, so it's important to know the different ways your body can express them.

If you aren't experiencing orgasms, look at your physical and mental health, as well as your current relationship environment. Have you had any illnesses that may have impacted your sexual health? Are you on any medications that may be impacting your arousal? Certain medications like antidepressants have been known to suppress arousal levels and one's ability to reach orgasm. If this applies to you, it may be worth

---

33 Michael Castleman, "The Most Important Sexual Statistic," *Psychology Today* (March 16, 2009), https://www.psychologytoday.com/us/blog/all-about-sex/200903/the-most-important-sexual-statistic.

a conversation with your medical provider to see if you have an alternative option for medication.

If you have a current sexual partner, do you feel safe enough to let yourself go there in your relationship? Desire is a strong influencing factor on whether or not you can bring yourself to orgasm with a partner. Trust is another factor, since an orgasm can be a vulnerable experience.

If you're having difficulties orgasming, it's totally worth taking a step back and asking yourself if you're in the right place to start having sex with a new partner. Going slowly and holding space for yourself is a great way to build desire. Make room and meet your physical body and mental outlook where it currently is. The more you are able to look inward and figure out what it takes to get you into the orgasm mindset, the more likely it is you'll be able to articulate your specific needs to your partner. Research suggests that while, yes, there is a large disparity between different genders when it comes to the frequency of orgasm during partnered sex,[34] individuals are usually able to reach orgasm more easily through masturbation. So paying attention to what you like during masturbation can help you express what you need and like to a partner, which is key to unlocking that team orgasm.

If you're masturbating and still unable to orgasm, it might be worth seeking out a sex therapist to better help you along your journey. Whether you have primary anorgasmia (you've never had an orgasm) or secondary anorgasmia (you've

---

34 Justin R. Garcia et al., "Variation in Orgasm Occurrence by Sexual Orientation in a Sample of U.S. Singles," *The Journal of Sexual Medicine* 11, no. 11 (November 1, 2014), https://doi.org/https://doi.org/10.1111/jsm.12669.

orgasmed before, but now you're unable to) they should be able to come up with a treatment plan.

Sex should be a time to de-stress, not stress yourself out, so be kind to yourself. Start with your desire and work your way up from there. Most importantly, try to enjoy the journey, and move away from thinking that orgasm is the destination.

LOW LIBIDO

Your libido is how you feel sexually—your sex drive or desire for sexual activity. Many outside factors can impact your libido, and regardless of your age, your libido can go up and down. Here are some of the most common factors that can affect it.

Stress

You're likely never without some form of stress in your life, but an overabundance can put a damper on your sex life. Try to see what you can take off your plate to lessen the burden stress puts on your relationship. Once you can free up some time, see if that helps put you back in the mood.

Lack of Satisfaction/Orgasm

If you aren't receiving the pleasure you want from your current sexual encounters, chances are that you aren't going to be eager to be intimate very often. If you find yourself in a place where you're faking your orgasms with your partner(s), take a step back and have an honest conversation with them about your likes and dislikes. Communication can improve your chances of satisfaction, which may in turn increase your desire for more sex.

Body Image

If you aren't feeling confident in your own skin, it may be hurting your levels of arousal. You may feel more reticent about how new partners will perceive you and just shut down the entire idea of sex before it even gets brought up. Try to see yourself through your partner's eyes and spend some time alone with your body. Consider making a gratitude list for your body, and feel free to refer to it whenever you're feeling like you're "less than." (See Chapter 6 for more tips on body image.)

Depression

If you're depressed, there is a high likelihood that it is impacting your sex life. Seek out a therapist to confirm the diagnosis and talk to them about steps you can take to help with the symptoms. Talk to them about your sex life as well, because some medications used in the treatment of depression can hinder your sex drive.

Poor Communication

If something is bothering you, speak up and talk to your partner about it. This is especially important if we're getting to know someone new. Silence breeds resentment and does nothing to help your sex life. Try to have these conversations outside of the bedroom and use "I statements" so it doesn't feel like you're attacking them. "I statements" are the opposite of blanket statements. "I statements" are usually specific and centered on you, rather than on the general thoughts, actions, or perceptions of another person.

An important part of using "I statements" effectively is taking responsibility for your own feelings and decisions.

These statements aren't about blaming or attacking your partner—that would defeat the purpose! For example, a great "I statement" might be: "I feel more in the mood for sex when I have more time in the evenings to relax. I need to work on ways to wind down and relax well before bedtime." An example of something that is NOT an "I statement" is: "I feel like you never help with cleaning up after dinner, and that's why I'm not in the mood for sex."

CHAPTER 6:

POSITIVE BODY IMAGE

WHAT IS BODY IMAGE?

Want to know a shocking statistic? When surveyed, only 4% of women in the world described themselves as beautiful.[35] Not only that, but 95% of American advertisements showcase a body type that only 5% of the population can naturally claim.[36] What?! When men were surveyed, they weren't so much concerned with fatness—rather they worried about the perceived lack of muscle.[37] Unless you completely live off the grid and don't consume media, there's no escaping the imagery and messaging put forth and its impact on our opinions of our own bodies.

---

35 Dove Research, "The Real Truth About Beauty: Revisited," Dove.com, last modified 2010, https://www.dove.com/us/en/stories/about-dove/our-research.html.

36 "Media and Body Image," The American College of Obstetricians and Gynecologists, last modified, 2016, https://www.acog.org/patientresources/faqs/especially-for-teens/media-and-body-image.

37 "Eating Disorders in Men and Boys," National Eating Disorder Association, last modified 2018, https://www.nationaleatingdisorders.org/learn/general-information/research-on-males.

This slow indoctrination toward hating our bodies starts when we're young. This self-hatred is supported by the subtleties of what is deemed attractive in society and strengthened during seemingly innocuous conversation. What many would call mindless brunch chatter can actually be the catalyst to a potential body-shaming scenario. Haven't seen a friend in forever? Congratulating them on how good they look and asking if they lost weight? Why is that the go-to standard? Do we have less value if we take up more space? Is this the luggage bin under the airplane? No. You are not luggage, so no bonuses if you happen to take up less space.

Think about it. Applauding moms for getting their body back. Assuming slim bodies are more "healthy." It's constant.

Other attributes like wrinkles, stretch marks, cellulite, grey hair, or saggy boobs can make people feel bad about the way they look. Society loves to tell you how to fix those things (at a price), promising it will make you feel better—but ultimately it's all about trying to sell you on products.

And even if we are exempt from criticism in our social lives, the media is nearly inescapable.

So what exactly is body image? Body image is your opinion about your physical form. Your feelings about how you look and exist in the world, and how you think other people see you, can range from positive to negative. Obviously, it's great when you love your own body, but it gets tricky when you aren't happy with what you see in the mirror. While avoiding the desire to attain society's standards of beauty is a topic that could fill a separate book, I'd like us to home in on what it means to have a healthy body image.

A healthy body image means that you accept and appreciate your body just as it is. Not letting the pressure of society sway your feelings may seem hard, but you can do it!

Positive body image isn't something you can just suddenly wake up and adopt, especially if it's a new concept for you. This may be a lifelong journey that you're working toward, and that's okay. Knowing that your value isn't tied to your physical form can help reframe your perception and boost your self-esteem. When you feel better, you leave space for more happiness, and I mean, who doesn't want that?

WAYS POOR BODY IMAGE HOLDS US BACK

When we don't feel good about our bodies, we put our life on hold. We say things like:

> *I'll buy that dress once I lose the weight.*
> *I'll wait until spring to take family photos.*
> *I'll start dating after _____.*

This is a terrible way to lead a life. Always in a state of pause. People who have poor body image can miss out on opportunities with friends, skip photos, have bad sex, fear aging, and contend with a host of other stressors that touch on every aspect of their lives. Getting a rein on negative body image is imperative to leading a more fulfilled life.

People can form resentments regarding their body shape and size, often citing it as the sole reason that they haven't met their desires or achieved happiness. Single people are particularly susceptible to this line of thinking, as they can lament over the idea that they are too fat, too old, too ugly to be searching for a partner.

> If only I were thinner, I would have . . .
> If only I had found a partner when I was younger, I
>   would have . . .
> If only I were taller, I could have . . .

We need to reframe our thinking to one of gratitude. Even if you've hated your body up until this point, you have to acknowledge that you're still here. This is the vessel that has carried you to this point in life. Also think about this: If we could hate our bodies into a shape we wanted, don't you think that would have worked by now? If you really take stock of all the good times you've had, you have to give your body credit for making them possible.

With gratitude, reframing your mindset, and recognizing abundance, you can start to help heal the rift between your conscious self and your physical body. According to Merriam-Webster, abundance is defined as "an ample quantity."[38] There is an ample quantity of a lot of things in our lives if we choose to see it. For a simple example of this, go outside and look at the grass (if you live in the frozen north like I do and it's winter, think snowflakes). There are so many blades! An abundance of blades! An abundance of love, friendship, new opportunities, and yes, even grass (or snowflakes) are around you all the time. Once you're able to recognize the abundance around you, you will have unlocked your consciousness to the possibilities.

I know it sounds woo-woo, but stay with me. You are a vital part of the world's abundance. You, in your body, with

---

38 Merriam-Webster, last modified September 21, 2020, https://www.merriam-webster.com/dictionary/abundance.

all of your gifts, can both contribute to and receive the abundance of the universe. Once you can shift your mindset into believing that you are in amongst the abundance, you will start to recognize it as it shows up in your life more and more. So the TLDR is: see it, believe it, receive it!

This isn't to say that there won't be some days when you struggle, but remember that your worth is more than what is on the outside!

HOW TO HONOR YOUR BODY

Give yourself permission to rest. We live in a go-go-go society, and our bodies need a chance to reset. Treat your body well by taking a luxurious bubble bath, getting a massage, or maybe just finding some time to lie in corpse pose on the floor (yoga's most relaxing position!). Consider this your permission slip to let your body rest without consequence.

Be mindful of the language you use when describing your body. Sadly, women are often the first to criticize themselves and find perceived flaws in their own appearance. We often sneak those criticisms into conversation in the form of a joke. But even if the negative comment was said in jest, you don't always know who was listening. Little ears are like sponges, and when they happen to hear someone they admire make a negative comment about their body or a body part, it can make them question their own worth. Something as innocuous as mentioning how you're skipping the fries because you went up a pants size, or mentioning that your new eye wrinkles make you look so ugly, can have a lasting impact on those who hear it. Even though you're saying it about yourself, someone may take what you said, internalize it, and find fault with the same things in themselves. This is especially troubling if you're saying disparaging things about yourself in terms of size around friends who are larger than you.

Remind yourself that society pressures us to be a certain way and that trying to live up to that expectation can be overwhelming at times. Lean on the support of your loved ones when you're feeling insecure or inadequate. They love you for who you truly are and not just for what you look like.

WHY DO WE HATE OURSELVES?

We hate ourselves because ads tell us that we need to fix our "problem areas." And it's not like it's just a few ads in one medium, it's everywhere. New Year's workout and diet plans making you think about spring break and needing a bikini body in just a few short months? They can be pretty compelling, but I'm here to save you the money and the time by dropping a secret.

Come closer.
Closer.
Do you have a body?
Good, then you have a bikini body! Wasn't that easy?

Companies rely on the will of the people, so if you're seeing some nonsense being advertised to you, call it out! With the power of social media, real change is actually available at the touch of the "post" button.

We have to ask ourselves who profits from this desire to make ourselves thinner or more attractive. Marketed with a sculpted ideal that few can attain, even the most innocuous ad can be quite provocative. If we aren't too careful, those airbrushed images and crafted messages can permeate our brains and make us question if we're good enough. That's why it's so vital to think critically about any media you consume.

Shows that feature major weight loss are just body shaming in the form of a contest. They want you to believe that happiness is just one modification away. You don't need to change something about yourself in order to have a great life, especially if you're only motivated to make that change for the sake of someone else. Make a change because you want it, not because you saw an ad or because someone asked you to.

Just because you know about someone's physical appearance, it doesn't mean that you know their history. Attributes like our genetic makeup, our cultural background, and our lifestyle are all varied, so it's a pointless exercise to compare yourself against someone who isn't you.

People of all body shapes and sizes deserve happiness and sexual satisfaction. As you begin to embrace who you are and the way you look, you'll find that you're happier in the long run. And the happier you are, the more confidence you'll have!

ELIMINATE NEGATIVE SELF-TALK

I strive to eliminate the negative self-talk in my head. It's taken a long time to fully love every part of myself, and it was hard won. Every now and then the voices of doubt come creeping back in, but I don't let them stay long. I am grateful and secure in my abilities, and I know that being kind to myself is the best thing I can do to achieve my goals.

For me, I love cooking and eating well. I have Post-it Notes with positive affirmations and reminders on them. Included are: "You are beautiful" and "Don't get caught up in the destination." I spend time with friends who can shake me out of any rut I may have fallen into, and I revel in the steadfast, unyielding love of my dog. I try to build and fortify this house of love, light, and joy, so that I may live in it, especially when the world makes me feel less.

Steps to Eliminating Negative Self-Talk in the Moment

Even with all of this knowledge in our back pocket, what if you come across a moment when those voices start to become loud again? Consider these steps:

▸ Take a breath.

▸ Breathe in and try to center yourself. Try to feel what is currently around you, and only what's around you in the moment. Bring your attention to your breath.

▸ Acknowledge your feelings about whatever is making you feel less worthy. Say them aloud to yourself or write them down. You are human! You cannot always control your thoughts, but you can control how you react to them. Feelings are normal—the good, the bad, and the ugly.

▸ Try to find out the root cause of where this insecurity is coming from: What is making your mind have a five alarm fire and spew unkind words? Are you worried about what your partner may think? Are you feeling less confident because you're comparing yourself to someone?

▸ Assure yourself by reframing the situation to reflect what the actual situation is. If you're feeling insecure with a new partner, assure yourself that they are with you because they like the whole you. Chances are they won't even notice your perceived insecurities unless you draw attention to them. You always have the right to slow things down if they're progressing quickly. (For more tips on how to reframe the situation, see the section below called "See Yourself as Your Best Friend Would.")

▸ Forgive yourself and vow to try to do better next time.

Eliminating negative self-talk isn't something that happens overnight. But with practice, we can help stop it in its tracks when it rears its head. And what you have worries or concerns over will change as your life goes on, but as long as you have a strong system in place, nothing will be able to fully uproot you from yourself.

BE THE BEST YOU

Single and confident people take care of themselves. I don't necessarily mean they live in the gym and buy kale by the pound, but rather they do what is best for them mentally and physically. They treat their body and spirit well, and they do it for themselves, not someone else.

And speaking of the body—do not get hung up on silly numbers on a scale or a tag. Those are not indicators of your worth in the world, nor should your happiness be contingent upon them. If you feel like you would like to make a physical change, begin working toward that change by agreeing to love yourself at the beginning of your journey and not just at the end. It is with that body that you are making a transformation, so be grateful about the place you're at now, and for the place you're going. Moreover, if you are kind to yourself, your body will show you what it wants to look like when it's happy and healthy.

Like we talked about earlier in our masturbation chapter, how you feel about your body is crucial to how you carry yourself in this world. People often think positive body image is waking up daily and saying, "Yes I love my body, I am perfect, amazing, wonderful." And while those are all great feelings to have about your body, it isn't necessarily the norm, and won't always feel true, especially not every day. We are constantly being barraged by society, our culture, our family, and at the end of the day ourselves, about why we look or don't look a certain way.

But even on the days when we feel less than "perfect, amazing, wonderful," we can still remind ourselves of the many ways in which our bodies bring us happiness and fulfillment. Our body is the one thing that is always with us as we traverse this world, so whether that is visiting beautiful places or hugging our loved ones, we need to be grateful. Appreciate the way our body brings us pleasure through our senses and allows us to access the joy that is in the world. Having a positive body image doesn't mean that you think you're perfect, or that you can't change it—it just means that you feel comfortable in your own body and grateful for how it serves you.

So before we get any further, I'd like you to take one minute to set a timer and apologize to yourself for all of the terrible-nasty-not positive-ugly-things you said about your body in the past.

Thank you for doing that.

This isn't an instant fix, but it is a step in the right direction to making peace with the skin that you live in. They say the grass is always greener on the other side. Looks can be deceiving because the grass is often fake. That's not my joke, but I saw the sentiment on a meme and I liked it and I took it.

Think about the top five people you admire. Your admiration doesn't necessarily have to be about their physical appearance. Just imagine those five people. Think about the reasons why you admire them. Maybe you think their life is perfect or they have everything going for them. And it might be true that they have a wonderful life, but I guarantee you they have their own struggles. Their own problems, concerns, and worries about themselves and their bodies. What you might love about them they might dislike about themselves, and that's why beauty is so subjective. Think about those characteristics that make you attracted to them. Do any of those apply to you? When you swap it and think about the things that might make people attracted to you, you can see that what one holds as precious can be anything.

SEE YOURSELF AS YOUR BEST FRIEND WOULD

This exercise will help you realize how aggressive we can be to ourselves. Here's a scenario: think about your best friend. They're feeling down. They say nothing looks good on them. They hate that their hair is thin, and they can't fit in any of their pants from the summer.

Would you say, "Yeah I was going to mention that. It sucks that you can't fit in your pants anymore." Or would you say, "None of that shit matters because I like you for you!" Hopefully you picked the latter response.

Anytime you have not kind thoughts about yourself, think about the advice you have recently given, or in that story example, the advice you would give to your best friend, and then give that advice to yourself. We are notoriously our own worst critics, and sometimes it takes reframing how we feel about ourselves to break through that ugly reductive logic.

Your friends are not your friends just because you look pretty. They love you for the whole you, and that should be front of mind any time that you feel not good about yourself. And as always, this isn't to say that you don't get to have bad days. I've been doing this work for years, and still some days I wake up and think I look like a hot mayonnaise sandwich (read: gross). One of the foundational beliefs behind positive body image is that you have the permission and the flexibility to feel your feelings, but you also have the wherewithal and systems in place to know that this feeling is fleeting, temporary, and not reflective of your true worth.

THE F WORD

I'm fat.

Right? If you don't know the answer to that, look me up! I'm sure that if I were to say that statement to many of you, your responses would look something like this:

No you're not!
You're not fat, you're beautiful!
Real women have curves.
Stop being so self-deprecating.

There is a fear around the word fat. Saying that I'm not fat, but I'm beautiful makes it seem like the two are mutually exclusive. I am a fat person. But we don't like that word so much that we've developed words that mean the same thing, but sound less aggressive. Words like:

- Plus size
- Husky
- Thicc
- Queen size
- Fluffy
- Above average
- BBW
- Cozy

While it's okay to use whatever language you're comfortable with, let's talk about the reality. It all means fat. And when we say fat, I think a lot of apprehension comes from the fear that someone won't like that you're fat.

Fatness should not be the reason that you decide to hold off on dating. If someone is after you just for your body, it won't be a lasting relationship anyway. You are so much more than your physical form, and the right person will realize that. Find a partner who enjoys all that you are and doesn't make you feel insecure about your body.

MIRROR EXERCISE

In order to make peace with your body, consider looking at it in the mirror. I know that can be confronting for some people, but avoidance isn't the way we start to heal the relationship we have with our bodies. Look at yourself naked (or as clothed as you'd prefer) in the mirror, pump up your favorite jams, and try to take stock of yourself objectively. Focus on what you like and consider why. With the risk of sounding like a hippy, it's time we stop judging ourselves on whether or not we are "normal" and time to start loving our diversity, because diversity is normal.

We are notoriously our own worst critics, and those inner critical voices can be crippling at times. Don't get stuck at looking at what you don't like. See it, acknowledge it, and then move on. Whenever a negative thought crosses your mind, try to follow it up with something positive. That might look something like this:

Oh great, I see my mustache is back. (negative and defeating)

My lips look good from all of the water I've been drinking. (positive and uplifting)

Continue to do this exercise and reveal more and more of what you love about yourself in the mirror. This isn't to get you a place where you look in the mirror and you absolutely love everything you see (although, wouldn't that be great?). This exercise is to help you realize that your body is enough, and worthy for whatever you want to pursue right now.

NORMALIZATION OF BODIES

How often are we plagued with the worry that we might not be normal? It's a common question that is posed not just in the sexological sense, but in everyday life as well.

According to Merriam-Webster, *normal*, in the context many are concerned about, is defined as "occurring naturally."[39] Despite the definition, *normal* is still a loaded

---

39 Merriam-Webster, last modified 2020, https://www.merriam-webster.com/dictionary/normal.

word. As we grow out of our youth, many of us realize that most of the concerns we had when we were younger are trivial now, but I think it is important to mention that sometimes concerns about whether we're "normal" can stay with us throughout our lives.

It is no wonder that so many people have bodily and sexual concerns—society shows us what is "normal" through curated, altered, and unnatural images, and when we do not measure up, the self-doubt begins.

Learning to love yourself in our current culture is tough, but not impossible. It also doesn't happen overnight. The first step on the journey is to decide that enough is enough, and you want to shift into a place where hate isn't welcome in regard to your body. This doesn't have to be some grand gesture either. It can be as simple as vowing to yourself that every time you look in the mirror and have something unkind run through your mind, you'll acknowledge it, but then follow it up with something that you do like about yourself, using the Mirror Exercise from earlier.

And if we're talking about bodies, we have to talk about ethnicity and racism. Racism can absolutely contribute to body image issues. Specifically, I can think of how hard the scrutiny was on Lizzo when she was just out there living her best life. Then people started the old trope of health trolling and equating fatness with diabetes. It was eye-rolling and exhausting. But, back to POC and feeling good about our bodies. Curate your social media feed. Look at the accounts you're following. Do they make you feel empowered? Beyond size, other facets like hair style and skin color can contribute to added dissatisfaction for nonwhite people. So be mindful of who you're following and what is being reinforced on the daily. Delete and add new accounts as necessary because what you surround yourself with influences you, no matter how immune you may think you are to those images. Any time we think certain kinds of bodies from diverse backgrounds are "supposed" to look a certain way, we are just shoving more people out of the proverbial box of happiness. Bodies from all kinds of ethnic backgrounds have different shapes and sizes.

Healing from this kind of systemic issue takes time, and you need to have forgiveness factored into this journey. It can be a lifelong one. Especially with mainstream media highlighting one specific kind of body type and constantly inundating you with products, pills, and programs to shame you into changing your body.

Give yourself permission to have bad days along this journey. There will be days when you feel absolutely yuck about yourself, and that's normal. You're human. Just know that those days will become fewer and fewer as you progress toward healing your body image, and hopefully one day loving the skin that you're in.

Here's how this can look IRL:

It's date number four, you're deep into a heavy make-out session, and clothes start coming off. Your date removes their shirt and you're practically drooling. You are so excited that you get to be with them. They move to help you take off your shirt, and then you freeze-frame. You have some apprehension about revealing yourself to your date, and the negative self-talk gets ready to stream across your mind like a news ticker. But you change the channel and tune back into your partner, focusing on what you like about them and the sensations they're creating in you. You remember that you are awesome, deserving of touch and sexual satisfaction, and that your date is excited to be with you. You imagine I'm on your shoulder cheering you on. Unfreeze frame. You happily lift your arms, let them take your shirt off, and continue as you were.

COMPLIMENTS UNRELATED TO APPEARANCE

Quick! Think of a compliment. Write it below:

_____

_____

_____

_____

Was this a compliment in regard to something you can see? In other words, was it a physical compliment? If this wasn't a physical compliment, great job! If it was, don't feel bad—it becomes a habit to compliment people's physical appearance.

It's easy to say something like, "Wow I love your hair." Now, this isn't an inherently wrong compliment, but I want to challenge you to go deeper when you're thinking of ways to boost those around you. Compliment people on something that is beyond the obvious, something people cannot see from the outside. This goes doubly for children, who, with their sponge-like minds and listening ears, are learning what to value about themselves based on your compliments.

I have compiled fifteen sentences for you to use on people in your life. You don't need to use these verbatim. Play around with the meanings and find one that fits the situation.

You inspire me.
You have a great laugh.
You light up the room.
I love your passion.
You are brave.
Your point of view is so refreshing.
You are doing important work.
You make me feel comfortable enough to be myself.
You're such a good listener.
Our conversations always make me feel better.
I never get tired of being around you.
I'm so happy that you're in my life.
The world needs more people like you in it.
I hope we know each other for a long time.
I value the time we spend together.

Once you've mastered these compliments and tried them out on your loved ones, turn them around and say them to yourself, too! What nonphysical qualities would you compliment about yourself?

BOPO FOOD

Think of the most decadent thing you've ever eaten. Like a brownie sundae. Something rich and sweet, ooey and gooey. What other descriptors came to mind? How long until you thought of the adjectives naughty or off-limits? If you didn't, bravo! But for everyone else, where did we get this idea that something created for enjoyment should be relegated to the naughty section? #JusticeForCakes!

It's nearly impossible to move through society without seeing some messages regarding the foods that we're putting in our mouths. From the "clean juice" shops to skinny drops, someone somewhere is trying to cash in on our insecurities. People pass a moral judgment on the foods you're consuming (better not be fat and eating a cheeseburger!), and that's especially exacerbated if your body falls outside the spectrum of what's deemed most attractive.

You can't tell the health status of someone just by looking at them. Health is not determined by weight and shape. And mental health is a key component of overall health: when you feel good, you can do more of what brings you joy. Try your best to fuel yourself with foods that satisfy you, but also allow yourself to live. For more on how to separate the ideas of weight and health, I recommend *Health At Every Size: The Surprising Truth About Your Weight* by Linda Bacon. I also love the book *Things No One Will Tell Fat Girls: A Handbook for Unapologetic Living* by Jes Baker.

The next time you eat something, try to think about how the food is going to fuel you rather than worrying about the calorie count. Your body needs sustenance, so try shifting your mindset to recognize the positives of food. This can help you avoid assigning a moral value to what you consume. Remember that bodies change, and any weight fluctuations you may experience aren't reflective of your worth. Diets don't work, especially those with severe calorie restrictions, so just skip them all together. Restrictive eating often swings like a pendulum into binge eating, and that isn't great for you either. Simple rule: eat when you're hungry.

When it comes to food, you should be thinking about it as nourishment. Your body needs fuel to survive. And definitely stop with the "good food"/"bad food" distinction. There are no bad foods, just consequences. If I just pound

Skittles (which are delicious) and chase them with root beer (which I also love), I'm probably not going to feel that great. Eating some Skittles might have been pleasant, but probably not in that amount. Likewise, I may start my summer mornings off with a kale smoothie because I have a kale garden and it makes me feel energized! Nothing inherently good or bad about it.

Don't think of food as a reward either. Again, food is what our body needs to survive, so if it's tied to your productivity, a number on a scale, or otherwise "earning" it, that's an unhealthy way to look at it. The right foods will be different for everyone, so don't compare yourself to someone else.

When it comes to exercise, I love to have people frame it as moving your body in a way that makes you happy. Exercise in a way that brings you joy. Maybe that means dancing, riding a bike, hiking a beautiful trail, taking your dog for a walk, tending an orchard. We want to frame exercise as a way to celebrate our bodies, not beat them down until they're into a shape that pleases us.

On a more specific note, if you are looking to make a change in your diet because of your health reasons, that is fantastic. Many of us make changes to our diet and lifestyle based on specific health concerns. But for those who look in the mirror and hate what they see, I have a message for you. You are exactly the size and shape you are supposed to be right now. Whatever your life path has been, this is where you ended up, so start loving yourself now. Not later, but immediately. We've all heard it, now embrace it: make peace with your own skin. Purge those negative thoughts right now! Remember that self-confidence can create success in all realms: career, personal happiness, relationship satisfaction, and beyond.

Food is the nourishment that we need to intake daily to exist. That's all. But a hunger for happiness can be found if we start to change our attitude around food. So the next time you say, "I'll be good today," at brunch with friends, let's hope it just means that you're going to tip well.

JAPANESE ONSEN ANECDOTE

In 2013, I was still riding the high of graduating from graduate school and knowing that I had done the work to finally call myself Dr. Megan Stubbs, Sexologist. Without going into too many details, let me just say that getting a graduate degree in sex is unlike any other degree path out there. Aside from the obvious learning of the sexual practices, we also did a lot of work with ourselves (no, not just masturbation!): mental work, confronting work, body image work.

It's not as easy as waking up one morning and deciding to suddenly be in love with yourself. You have to do the work to understand where your feelings are coming from, unpack all of the messages you've been bombarded with from the media, family, and friends. At the time, that sector of my education was ongoing.

In the spring of that year, I experienced my first Japanese onsen, or hot spring. While using the onsen, you are not allowed to wear any clothing. This is quite the liberating experience, especially when you go with family members—for me that included my sister, mother, grandmother, and great aunts. Are you really living if you haven't seen your family members naked? Our ages spanned from eighteen to eighty-three! Obviously, it is not polite to stare considering that everyone is naked, but you're bound to look around.

While I was submerged in the hot and mineral-rich water,

I took in the scene around me. There were over one hundred women in the facility at the time, and something struck me as very peculiar as I was surveying all of the bodies. Even for those with lean and lithe builds, I noticed almost every woman had stretch marks. Even with all the schooling and personal work I had done, it was at this moment when a particular category of self-love really hit me: stretch marks can happen to anyone.

Stretch marks are a type of scarring that can happen when there is rapid growth and stretching of the skin. They often occur during puberty, pregnancy, or even muscle building. The marks can appear anywhere on the body, but are usually found in areas where there are high amounts of fat stored, like the abdomen, breasts, arms, thighs, hips, and buttocks. Stretch marks are commonly a darker, reddish color, which later fade into a lighter hue over time. The dark color is from the dermis (the inner layer of skin) being torn and exposing the blood vessels in the skin. As the tears heal, the stretch marks return to a color similar to the surrounding skin. They pose no health risks but can often cause mixed feelings to those who have them.

Since my experience in the onsen, there has been an amazing movement of women proudly declaring they love their stretch marks and/or other scars. I, like many women, cheered and applauded the movement. Although, I began to see a common tone from many of the messages about women loving their stretch marks: It was always a story surrounding motherhood. I still cheered with them, but it made me pause.

What about those of us who have not experienced pregnancy and childbirth? Are our triumphs over fighting beauty standards less valid because we don't have a story beyond our bodies changing super rapidly, and that's it? I personally don't have a child to show off proudly as the reason for my scars. I can tell you about my unyielding love of cheese, but somehow I thought that paled in comparison. Maybe your story is that puberty came on like a freight train and this is what happened. Whatever situation or circumstance happened—pregnancy, illness, puberty, weight gain, or something else—let me say to you that it is completely valid and part of your story; your unique story.

The largest sexual organ on our body is our skin, and when there are perceived flaws on it, it can be the source for many negative thoughts. The prevalence, let alone the normalcy, of stretch marks should be widely known. In no way are they an indication of damaged goods. And if you see a person without them and feel jealous, remember: another person's beauty is not the absence of your own.

Take the challenge and embrace yourself for all that you are. You are more than the sum of your scars and imperfections. Your newfound confidence will shine brighter than the appearance of lines on your skin!

TEACHING SEX CLASSES ON A CRUISE

Being a sexologist comes with many unexpected job perks. I have had the privilege of teaching sexuality classes to adults at resorts and on cruise ships. Now while this may seem like all fun and games, there is actually a serious takeaway from my schedule. At any time of year, we're being constantly bombarded with messages about our body. If it's winter, we're hearing about holiday weight. If it's the New Year, it's the "New Year, New You." If it's springtime, it's spring break or preparing for that bikini body/beach body. It never ends.

Vacationing, especially in a tropical location, can really make you think about your body. If you're not in hot weather clothes, you stand out. On these vacations of adult nature, bodies are usually at the forefront, and here's something surprising: I saw all iterations of bodies. The people who were on vacation were there to enjoy themselves and not be held down by societal norms around what a good body is. Now this is easy to say, but not something that is as easy to implement.

You may think that you've been exposed to it all, or seen everything, but I challenge you to attend a lifestyle event and tell me that everything you see is old news. Here at these gatherings you are going to see old bodies, young bodies, skinny bodies, fat bodies, wrinkly bodies, stretch mark bodies, hairy bodies, dark skin, light skin, disabled bodies, and more. And they're all having fun. No one is letting the shape of their body get them down. In fact, they sometimes play it up!

And here is where the bonus round comes into play: they're having sex! Well, not all of them, but many have taken a romp in the red room, and the pool parties are by no means rated PG either. There is something very human about watching other humans have live sex in front of you. There is an authenticity that cannot be found in pornography. Of course, some people are there to put on a show for you, but when you strip people down to their bare skin and watch how they give and receive pleasure, it's something special. You have an inner feeling of peace about your own body and what you do with it. It's difficult to put into words adequately.

If you'd like to explore these kinds of environments, look for lifestyle friendly resorts, clothing optional places, or even host your own with a group of friends!

CHAPTER 7:

DATING
WANT LONG–TERM ,
HAVE SHORT–TERM CONNECTIONS

O ne of the most challenging things someone who is looking for a long-term relationship has to contend with is all of the false starts and short-term connections that don't lead anywhere. Unfortunately those are all part of the process. You have to start somewhere, and until it ends, you won't know if it is a short-term or long-term connection. But after your fifth false start, it can totally feel daunting or not even worth the effort. I hear you! Try to find good takeaways while traversing this space, and appreciate those people with whom you have short-term connections, whatever they may bring to your life. Stay present and enjoy the time getting to know someone new.

HOW TO MEET PEOPLE IN THE WILD

Where is the place to meet other single people? Clearly the internet is an ocean of options with all of the dating apps available, but what about foraging in the wild? Here are some places you can look for a date in real life.

School

This is an easy one since you already have something in common! It can be easy to find someone in your program or that you happen to see on the regular. You may have a little bit of data on them, from how they act in class or who their friends are, so give it a try!

Gym

This is a great place to meet someone who shares this activity with you. There are lots of opportunities to make an interaction happen. Ask for help, maybe a spot, or catch their eye in the mirror. Also, keep in mind that some people are at the gym, just to be at the gym and not to meet anyone. Use your best judgment.

Coffee Shop

Your local barista is the keeper of so much knowledge. Let them know you're on the hunt for someone. Their job is to get to know their clientele, and they might be able to act as your designated wing person. Maybe you're not at your local coffee shop—does that mean you can't find someone? No! If you find yourself out in public and catch the eye of someone you're interested in, ask them to watch your stuff while you go to the bathroom. Then when you get back (assuming they haven't stolen your laptop), you can thank them and strike up a conversation.

Walking Your Dog

Honestly, using your pet is the best cover to meet someone. They are the ultimate wing person. They are a magnet for people of all types, and you can easily strike up a conversation with someone who came over to greet your four-legged friend.

ONLINE DATING

The phrase *online dating* can raise a whole host of reactions and emotions. Some say it is the way of the future, and others believe that it is responsible for ruining true human connection. While you can passively be a single person, there's something to be said about actively signing up for an online dating site. It's like you're really owning your singleness.

Regardless of how you feel, you cannot deny that technology is responsible for bringing together a wide range of people that would otherwise not have the opportunity to meet. If online dating is something that might be in your near future, all of the options can be a little daunting. With some basic information, safety tips, and an open mind, you will be a pro in no time.

Now, before you start traversing the digital world of singles, here are some important tips to keep in mind:

About Me

Write something unique. Who doesn't like to travel, laugh, or hang out with friends? Try to say something that is specific to you. Play up your assets and self-promote. Leaving out what you're interested in or good at can make you come off as dull. At the same time, leave a little mystery. And as a general rule, don't write anything that you wouldn't tell someone on the first date. They don't need to know about the six cats you have at home.

Photo

Make sure your first profile photo is of your face. No group photos. They'll assume the worst and quickly move on—nobody wants to search through a series of pictures to figure out which person you are. No cropped photos with your ex's face awkwardly chopped off. We can always tell, or we will always wonder who that used to be. Try not to leave your profile with just one photo either. That can come off scammy. This is your chance to show off different facets of your life. Hit them with the main best headshot and then use the other photos as a chance to show off some activities you like or some experiences you've had. And remember, no photos with exotic animals: #TigerKing.

What Are You Looking For?

If you feel the need to specify what you're looking for, consider staying away from negativity. Phrases such as "Don't message me if you still live in your parent's basement," or "Don't bother if you weren't born before 1985" make you seem shallow.

Online dating may seem a little daunting and awkward at first, but it gets better as you develop your interest level and dating style. It's fine to take a break from online dating, and it's completely normal to get discouraged at times. It's an unfortunate fact that we even have to name the practice of ending all communication with no warning whatsoever—ghosting—because it happens so frequently in the online dating environment. But if an online match "ghosts," take it with a grain of salt and move onto the next one. Wondering about the motives or reasons why they stopped contacting you won't get you anywhere. The reasons could have nothing to do with you, and you'd still be in the same position whether you knew or not.

My most important message with dating of any kind is that if a date isn't going well, you are permitted to leave. It's something that took me years to learn. It may look bad on the surface, but *you don't owe them anything.* Not even if they paid for your drinks or your two scoops of ice cream.

In addition, always have a safe call. A safe call is someone that you trust, with whom you share the details of your date. They should be actively waiting for you to let them know you are safe. So tell a friend who you're meeting and where you're going, and have a check-in time for after the date. You can even have a preprogrammed mid-date call just to make sure things are going okay. This can be a great way to end a date that is going poorly. "Oh sorry, I have to leave! My friend needs help watering her plants!"

"CHECK PLEASE" ANECDOTE

I was a young Megan working at a coffee shop when I met a guy who worked at a nearby store chain. As he came into the coffee shop more and more often, we slowly got to know each other. Eventually the mutual interest led us to make our first date.

We decided on sushi downtown. The day arrived, and I chose to wear a nice sundress. The place we were going was not formal by any means, but if it's summer, I'm in a sundress, so here we are. I drove downtown, parked in a parking ramp, and made my way to the restaurant. We agreed to meet at 7:00 p.m., and I went to look at my phone in my purse, but it wasn't there. I'd left it in my car. Was I going to walk back all the way just to get my phone, when I was about to have a date filled with conversation and no phone time? Absolutely not, so I continued on my way. I was the first to arrive. I said, "Table for two, please," and I sat down to wait.

And wait.

And wait.

Let me tell you about the exponentially building level of discomfort from knowing that you're being stood up. It is not a good feeling. I knew I should have brought my phone. I played mental games with myself for twenty-five minutes before I got up and left. I swear all eyes were on me. (I was hot.) I made it back to my car, snatched up my phone, and saw I had two missed text messages from him.

Text 1: Yo
Text 2: Yoooooooooooooooooooooooooooo

I wish you could have seen my nonplussed face. This was only the foreshadowing of even worse times ahead.

I asked where he was. He said he was "at the spot." He was most definitely not at the spot, as I had just spent twenty-five embarrassing minutes by myself at the fucking spot. I asked him which restaurant he was waiting at. He texted the name, and the two restaurants both started with the same letter, but one was clearly downtown (where I was!) and the other was NOT downtown. I wish you could see my face as I'm writing this.

I was like, okay, innocent mistake (he was hot, so he got way more slack than he deserved). I drove to the other restaurant to meet him. I wasn't going to waste an outfit. I should have just hit the Taco Bell drive-thru and gone home.

I arrived at the restaurant and scanned the tables for him. No need because this is what he shouted, so everyone including me could spot him.

Him: AYE YO! I'M HERE IN THE CORNER!
wildly gesticulates with his arm

I should have left.

Instead, I headed over to the table to sit with him. Now, I'm not some clotheshorse and I did say this was a casual restaurant, but what in the actual fuck was he wearing? I'll tell you.

He was in his running shoes, tear-away pants the likes of which I haven't seen since middle school, a shirt with the sleeves cut off, and a snapback hat, on backwards. I was slowly dying on the inside.

He told me he ran to the restaurant (very eco-friendly of him, but this is a date bro). He asked if I wanted to do a sake bomb. I declined.

I sat there as he beat the table until his shot of sake fell into his pint of beer. I now see that scene as a metaphor for how the date was going. I was going to go drown myself later in the river. Kidding!

When our server came to take our order, I ordered three sushi rolls and he said, "DAMN YOU EAT A LOT!" I literally cannot make this up. That statement caught some unfriendly eyeballs from both the server and me.

In anticipation of our sushi, he decided to crack open his set of chopsticks early and proceeded to rub them together so forcefully that I had an out-of-body moment, imagining we were on *Naked and Afraid* and we needed to start a fire.

Rubbing your chopsticks together is highly rude in Japanese culture (this dude would have never been introduced to grandma), and it was just another tally in the "never again" chart in my head.

What we talked about was inconsequential and clearly forgettable. I do remember one last sake bomb on his part, and him asking if I'd like to go back to his place. I declined and never went out with him again!

Moral of the story, I know that dating can be hard, and not all first dates are great! Some can be downright nightmares, and that's why I urge you to leave if you feel uncomfortable. But never forget them! These dates will remind you to never take a great partner for granted.

TRAITS OF A GREAT PARTNER

That's easy! He should be tall, dark, and handsome. Wait, that was only three. He also should have a flashy car and a huge . . . bank account. Done! Hello, dream lover. (Cue the record scratch.) For those of us who reside in the real world, it takes more than just superficiality to make us consider a partner for a long-term relationship. While it takes many different traits for a relationship to work, the traits listed below seem to be universal in healthy, happy, and successful relationships.

Having a solid idea of what you are looking for can better help you recognize it in the wild. Whether this is for short- or long-term relationships, having a baseline expectation of what you're looking for can help you differentiate whether or not someone is worthy of you and your time.

They Are Loyal

A supportive partner is one who stands by you through good times and bad. When the bad times do come, they are the first one to step up next to you and help battle whatever life obstacles come your way. This is someone who you can trust and rely upon no matter what the situation is. Their commitment to you and your relationship is paramount, and they will do everything within their power to create happiness and success.

They Challenge You

This isn't someone who is argumentative, but rather someone who challenges you to progress. We all have the propensity to become complacent from time to time, and our partner should notice our lulls and help get us back on track. This kind of partner supports you and embraces your desire to grow. They have a genuine care to see you succeed and have the wherewithal to tell you when you can do more. They want to see you go out into the world and get what you deserve.

They Inspire You

Sometimes life is difficult, and you can feel like all of your options have been attempted, but a partner who inspires you can reignite your flame. This is someone who can reach you on a deeper level and help you reflect on who you are as a person. When you have this kind of support at home, the sky's the limit. You can develop insights that you never thought of before.

They Initiate Intimacy

With many relationships, in the beginning everything is hot and heavy. As time goes on, the initial lust and new relationship energy (NRE) transforms into something less blazing, but still hot nonetheless. A partner who initiates intimacy is attracted to the person they met years ago, whether it was one year ago, five, or even twenty! Things like aging and motherhood can affect the way we view our bodies and sexuality, but a great partner doesn't let those aspects change the way they feel about us.

They Sacrifice for You

Has a partner ever put aside something for the advancement of the two of you? Has a partner ever said no to a career or travel opportunity because of you? This can be a strong indicator of someone's commitment to you. Don't expect them to put their life on hold, but allow them to make sacrifices if that is what they want to do. Pay attention when they do something for the progress of your relationship. Someone who is willing to drop everything and be by your side is someone special.

They Agree with You on Life Plans

This doesn't mean you make a death pact with them, but rather you both are on board for the same kind of life. You agree on certain things like finances, children, what city you will live in, whether you want pets (red flag if no. Kidding! But not really . . .), and more.

A great way to use this checklist is to first ask yourself: How well did you exude these traits in your previous relationships? Are there any areas that you need to work on yourself? Bringing awareness to yourself about whether you behave the way you wish to see partners behave is a great way to keep your future relationships healthy and happy.

Write down the traits you're looking for with a partner and then see if you can recognize them in someone you think has potential. There's no reason to settle with someone who doesn't make you happy or meet your standards. Remember, not every date has to turn into a boyfriend, and not every boyfriend has to be husband material. You are enough, and everyone deserves to have a great partner, whether they are a short-term or long-term partner.

DATING AGE CALCULATOR

When I was twenty-eight, I was active on the dating app scene. After exhausting people on my app who were within a few years of myself, I decided to expand that search in the older age range. I opened up my age parameters, and the new matches flooded in. I ended up matching up with this forty-two-year-old man. We started to talk, and it was really great. Things progressed, and we decided that it was time that we meet in real life and go on a date. Our first date was very nice, but something he said stuck with me till this day. He told me that one of the reasons he swiped right on me was because I was within the correct age range. I was confused. Like, did he mean that I fit within his parameters? No. He meant according to the age-range calculator. To find your limits, you apply this math:

Lowest age = Your current age divided by two, plus seven years

Highest age = Your current age multiplied by two, minus seven years

So what he was saying was that if I were twenty-seven, he would have swiped left on me! This is worth checking out when looking for what age ranges you should be pursuing, but it is not by any means a hard rule. There are many people who have found happiness with people they share large age gaps with.

HOW YOU SABOTAGE YOUR NEW RELATIONSHIP

I'm not sure what to call this, but it's that time when you stop being on your best behavior. When you start to think things are implied. You stop using please and thank you. You don't show as much gratitude as you would if a friend did something for you. Yes, your partner is someone who is in your corner, but that doesn't mean that they don't still appreciate your gratitude. When they pick up the bill. When they bring you back a drink from the bar. When they open the door for you. When they pack your lunch. It's the little things that count.

Also, unchecked jealousy can be a threat to a new relationship. Jealousy is sometimes unavoidable, but if you let it fester without communicating feelings, resentment can build and become a recipe for disaster. Communicate your feelings with your partner instead of making assumptions.

I know I've talked a lot about communication, but it's a habit that never goes out of style in a relationship. Unless you're a mentalist who knows what your partner is thinking, you need communication. Try to show your appreciation for them daily—show them with your actions as well as your words. It doesn't have to be some grand gesture; the little things are important too. And when you fight, because it's bound to happen, keep in the back of your mind that it isn't you v. your partner, it is your partner and you v. the problem.

PRE-DATE RITUALS

If it's been a while since you've been on a date, be your own best hype person and get excited. This is a great way to work out any pre-date nervousness and just feel good about yourself.

Here are some things to try before your next date:

In the shower: Skip the loofah or washcloth and use your hands! Lather up skin on skin, and truly feel yourself by caressing all of your parts. Revel in the tactile sensation and imagine it's your date, or your celebrity crush.

Music: Blast the songs that make you feel sexiest. Bonus points if you do it while in the shower. Playing your favorite sexy songs while dancing naked always help boost the mood and confidence.

Audiobook/podcast: Have some sexy stories playing in the background as you get ready. I might recommend you check out Dipsea or the Literotica Podcast. Who knows, you may just hear some tips that you can use on your date that same night.

Fantasize: A fun mind trick you can employ is thinking about a past sexy experience. Play out your dream fantasy in your head and be super detailed about it. Incorporate all of your senses into the memory. How did it feel, what did you see, what did it sound like, how did it taste? I'm getting turned on already!

Bonus move: Taking on a sexy alter ego can be a playful way to up your sexy factor. I know that when I wear a particular shade of red lipstick, I become a sexier version of myself. MAC Ruby Woo FTW.

MASTURBATE BEFORE A DATE

Who doesn't get a little nervous before a first date? Hands up please. No one? Right.

Even if you're the most charismatic, confident, good-looking person out there, you may still feel a little uncertainty in your mind. Is masturbating the new pre-date Ωactivity to help alleviate those nerves? Most of us have seen that scene from *There's Something About Mary*.

All joking aside, is this a viable option to cure a case of the nervies? Well, it might help to put you in a more relaxed or happy state.

But can a pre-game O help keep your mind off sex on your date? I'm highly doubtful. If you're concerned with thinking about sex the entire time on your date, I don't think masturbation will help keep you out of the mental sheets. If you're with your date and things are progressing nicely, and you're attracted to them, you probably are going to think about sex. AND THAT'S OKAY! We are sexual beings. Your date isn't going to be able to read your mind, and as long as you don't whip off the tablecloth and take them right there on the table, you'll be fine.

Masturbation and orgasm have no bearing on the level of your sex drive. When you orgasm, your body relaxes and releases tension in your muscles. You get an overall feeling of well-being and calm. But also keep in mind, a simple orgasm won't quell your sex drive completely. Just think of an orgasm as a quick, free, fun release that can help put you in a better mindset; pre-gaming.

What can we take home from this? Can an orgasm help take sex off the brain? Nah. Can an orgasm help alleviate some nervousness or stress? Absolutely an orgasm can help. So when you're getting ready for your date, picking out your perfect outfit, and doing your hair just so, take some time for yourself and tap into your built-in stress reliever. An orgasm a day can keep the nervies away.

WHAT TO CARRY IN YOUR PURSE

For those readers who carry a purse, when heading out on a date, I want you to channel your inner Girl Scout. Always be prepared. You never know what life is going to throw at you, so it can be great to have supplies to combat a curveball.

Money: This should be obvious, but don't leave home without money. This can come in handy for food, drinks, or even money for a ride home.

Tissues: These are handy if you have a runny nose or the only single bathroom in the entire restaurant is out of toilet paper (#ToiletPaperGate2020).[40] Tissues have saved me so many times.

Lip balm: It's always good to have this on hand. Both to keep your lips hydrated and to keep them ready for any potential kissing action.

---

40 Marc Fischer, "Flushing out the True Cause of the Global Toilet Paper Shortage amid Coronavirus Pandemic," *The Washington Post*, last modified April 7, 2020, https://www.washingtonpost.com/national/coronavirus-toilet-paper-shortage-panic/2020/04/07/1fd30e92-75b5-11ea-87da-77a8136c1a6d_story.html.

Mints: Maybe you just ate some aggressively flavored dinner and that little Andes mint was not enough to freshen your breath. Keeping a tin of these in your purse is easy, and you can always offer your date one.

Phone charger: Historically this is not a common purse requirement, but in this day and age, when our phones are our lifelines, it's always good to have access to power. This can be especially useful if you find yourself in a different part of town and you need to get a ride home. No one wants the anxiety of seeing 2% battery while they're waiting for their Lyft.

Condoms: You never know where the night will take you!

COMMUNICATION

Slide into DMs

Here are a few things to keep in mind if you want to slide into someone's DMs. First of all, prepare yourself that the person you're DM-img may not respond. The chance that they will respond significantly goes down if they have a huge following. Don't be that person who says hi, hi, hi, hey, fuck you you're ugly. Another thing to consider is the public/private status of your profile. If the person you're messaging can't see who you are and what you're about, they're probably going to think you're a stranger danger. As far as your message goes, be cool, be calm, and be authentic. Don't open up with something creepy or negative. Say your thoughts and then wait. Bonus points if you tie in your message to something they've recently shared.

Determine the Relationship Conversations

When people ask about you and the new person you're dating, what do you say? Are you dating? Are you exclusive? What is up, girlfriend? Have you had the "determine the relationship" conversation yet? When one person starts to develop more feelings AND they don't speak up, that's when some problems can arise. This can be a vulnerable time, but you don't know how they feel if you don't ask.

Be Cool

While this can seem like a critical turning point for your relationship, you have to be cool. Make sure some time has elapsed with the two of you together. You've gone out for a while and things have taken a natural progression. Then, bring it up in person. Don't make it weird and send a text that says something like "we need to talk." That's so anxiety inducing! Even when my best friend texts me that I hate it! And we aren't even dating!

Ultimatums

This is not the way to get your partner to be with you. You want to have someone be with you of their own free will, not because you forced their hand into a position. Just have a conversation with them. Say something like, "I've really enjoyed getting to know you over these last few months. I think we might have something together. Where are you at with this? Would you like to date exclusively?"

Be Prepared for All Responses

I always try to warn people about asking questions they don't want to know the answers to. If you aren't ready to hear about a potential rejection, it might not be the best time to ask about taking your relationship to the next level. But, that leaves you stuck where you are, and if you have growing feelings beyond what are being given to you now, that might leave you feeling sad. A "yes" is easy to understand—it's the rejection that we have to be prepared to cope with. You are absolutely able to talk to your partner about what's going on, but prepare yourself for the potential that they aren't in the same place as you, emotionally. And if that conversation shifts into an argument, it might be time to take a step back.

What Is Ghosting?

Ghosting is the act of ending a relationship by disappearing from someone's life (or messages) without any kind of contact or word that you're ending it. Ghosting is a really shitty way to end a relationship. It can leave people feeling hurt and confused, so do them the courtesy of saying, "Hey I don't think this is going to work out." It's the adult thing to do.

AM I SPENDING TOO MUCH TIME WITH THE PERSON I'M DATING?

I wish there was a magical rubric that told you how much quality time is "good" in a relationship, especially a new one, but alas, there is not. If you and the person you're dating are enjoying time together a lot, that's great! I would only be concerned that too much time is being spent together if you and/or your partner were ignoring your pre-existing relationships, like family or friends. A super red flag is if your partner tries to create a rift between your family and friends (hello "Dirty John").

If anything makes you feel gross, take a step back and

check in with a trusted friend and talk about the situation. But if not, enjoy your time together! New relationships are often high on NRE, so it's not a surprise that you want to spend every waking moment talking, connecting, or otherwise!

DATING RED FLAGS

The thing with red flags is that we know when they pop up. But the question is, do we listen to them when they do? What are they signifying in our life right now? Here are some common relationship red flags.

- You feel like you need to convince those around you that your relationship is great.
- Your friends don't like them. Your closest friends know you best and also want the best for you. If they are expressing some misgivings, listen to them. They may be able to see things you can't.
- You're comparing your relationship to others. You don't know what's happening in someone else's relationship. Relationships can look different in private, for celebrities and friends alike, so just do what's right for you and your partner. If there are attributes you see in other couples that you'd like to have in yours, have a conversation about it. But starting off with "Why can't you be more like *insert name of couple that seems to have it all together but likely has their own ish going on*?" isn't the best way to do so.
- You aren't talking about sex. Communication is key in all things. If you notice something, say something. Once you understand where your partner is coming

from, you can better form a plan of action in case things are at a mismatch. Assumptions really do nothing for us.

▶ The person you're dating is spending a ton of time on social media. Everyone has their thing (and who hasn't been sucked into the rabbit hole of cute puppy videos?), and if that's their hobby, that's okay! But! If it's becoming an issue (aka, they're spending all their time posting instead of getting back to you), talk to your partner about it. Having an open dialogue can help stave off those conversations that sound accusatory and help foster those that are seeking understanding. Social media is tricky, and I urge caution when equating "likes" outside of your relationship as a reflection of your own relationship happiness and status.

LONG-TERM POTENTIAL?

Are you wondering if this STR has the potential to become an LTR? While there are no required rules for relationships, many happy, successful couples do agree on a few certain aspects of their lives. They agree on their life plan together. This means that they have similar views on things like where to live and whether or not they want children. Couples generally need to agree on how they're spending their money. If this isn't part of an open conversation, a lot of resentment and arguments can result from lack of transparency.

I will say that couples 100% need to agree on their communication style. In addition to finding out each other's love language, it is imperative that you and your partner know how to communicate effectively. Whether it is to show that you care or to resolve a problem that has arisen, you need to make sure you're both in a place to share and comprehend.

A ride or die relationship is a relationship that has resiliency. The partnership is able to thrive in good times and bad. There is security in knowing that each partner can come to the other with anything and that they can work through it. They fight effectively and always keep the bigger picture (the relationship) in mind. Now with that being said, someone else's ride or die may not look like yours. That's what is so special about relationships. You are able to decide what terms work for you and your partner.

NRE: WHAT IT IS AND HOW TO MAKE IT LAST

New relationship energy is what people mean when they say they're drunk with love. When you have NRE, you're high on life and your partner. Everything you discover about them is exciting, and you can't wait to discover more.

To keep the NRE alive, never stop dating your partner. What that means is to continue to explore and make new memories with them. Try not to let complacency set in and dim your relationship's shine. That isn't to say that you have to be going on full throttle the entire time you're dating, but never take your partner for granted. Eventually, your relationship will transition into a space where it's okay that you aren't going spelunking and eating scorpions for dinner. You will be able to have your shared memories to sustain your relationship and move from infatuation to comfort and companionship.

FRIENDS WITH BENEFITS

FWB is a contentious topic. Many believe that it cannot work and has the potential to ruin your friendship. I don't like speaking in absolutes, and additionally, I don't believe that friends with benefits can't work. Why do I have this confidence? Because I have successfully had many friends with benefits relationships in my life. And guess what, we're still friends!

In order to have a successful friends-with-benefits situation, you have to have exceptional communication. Talk about your situation with your friend. Where is your mind at? Talk about the what-ifs. Be upfront about any boundaries you may have, and discuss your expectations around letting each other know if someone else is also in the equation. Talk about the communication frequency you two envision having, and if there are certain times not to hit each other up (you know, like a 2:30 a.m. "Are you up?" text).

Don't expect this relationship to transition into a dating relationship. If you are starting to have feelings for something more, let your friend know.

This is a casual arrangement, so that means it has the potential to end. It can end if either of you meet someone or it just stops being a good fit for you. And that's okay!

REJECTION

Nobody likes the feeling of rejection. We're far removed from our days of being selected last for the kickball team (maybe? Sorry if this is still happening with your adult league), but the thought of not being valued still hurts. Whether you're being selected last for kickball or someone you thought you had a great connection with isn't responding to your texts, it can leave you feeling down. This feeling can seem personal, when it isn't necessarily the case. Sometimes the rejection hurts so badly that it almost feels like a physical ache.

Interestingly, there was a study done at the University of Michigan that looked at this phenomenon.[41] Using functional magnetic resonance imaging, fMRI, the researchers devised an experiment that would bring about the feelings of rejection (for example, participants looking at a photo of an ex) and mapped the areas of the brain that were activated. They also devised a test that elicited physical pain (an arm zap) to the participants. In comparing both of the fMRI results, the areas of the brain that are responsible for processing physical pain were the same ones that lit up during the feelings of rejection. So no, you aren't crazy when rejection hurts!

When we're talking about rejection, we have to talk about the ways we process it. More specifically, how we treat ourselves after the experience. Ideally that would include talking to ourselves kindly, wrapping ourselves in a big hug, and saying, "Onto the next one!" In reality though, many people decide that this is the time to give themselves the dress down. All of the negative thoughts flood in:

I'm so stupid . . .
I can't believe I thought that . . .
Of course they said no, you're . . .
Who could love you with baggage like . . .

---

41 Ethan Kross et al., "Social Rejection Shares Somatosensory Representations with Physical Pain," *Proceedings of the National Academy of Sciences of the United States of America* 108, no. 15 (April 12, 2011): 6270–6275, https://doi.org/https://doi.org/10.1073/pnas.1102693108.

All of the horrible things that our brain can flash through in a few seconds. All of the belittling, self-critical, and self-destructive things.

Listen up! We don't need to kick ourselves when we're already down! Trying to shift our reactions and break away from this often default reaction is so important in traversing rejection.

Absolutely feel the feelings. You get to feel sad when rejection happens—that's natural. Chances are you're going to have many more throughout your life! The better able we are to navigate the post-rejection feelings, the better able we'll be to return to our normal state.

Trying to change any habit first requires you to recognize it. I'm a lip picker. There, I said it. It's out in the open now. I'm not just sitting here thinking, "Hmm, now would be a good time to pick my lips" and then diving in. It's sneaky! That's why it's a habit. Recognizing the behavior is the first step. If you don't know you're doing it, you won't know what to fix. Forgive yourself for saying the not nice things and tell yourself that you'll try to do better next time.

Dear Lips, I'm sorry I tried to pick the dry parts and put it in the skin box again. I will be more mindful about applying lip balm to keep you supple and crack free.

Once you've recognized it and put a stop to it, you can move onto the next step: Remember who the fuck you are! (See "Say it Loud, Say It Proud.") Remember all the reasons why you're a catch, an awesome person, worthy of love and having your desires met. This is so important!

That said, even if you recite all of the reasons why you're

kickass, you still might feel down. This is okay! Take this time to remind yourself of a time when you rejected someone. Remember how you were juggling so many things, or the timing wasn't right, or you just weren't feeling it? How often did you reject someone because they were absolutely a terrible person? Hopefully not that often—more often than not, I bet it was because they just weren't YOUR person. And that's okay! The same notion applies when you get rejected. It's really not you, it's them. Remember, you can be the juiciest peach in the basket, but if someone is like, "Well actually, I'm looking for a mango right now," then you still won't be the best fit. It's all good, just wait around for your peach eater (*insert gigantic wink face*).

It takes bravery to put yourself out there, so congratulate yourself on making moves! Just because someone said no to you doesn't mean that you should remove yourself from the dating pool. Rejection is a normal part of dating, and once you get more comfortable with it, you'll understand that it's less about who you are, and more about who your potential partner was at that moment in time.

CHAPTER 8

IMPORTANT CONVERSATIONS ABOUT HEALTH

Talking about your health and STI status is arguably one of the most important conversations you will have with a new sexual partner, followed by the crucial "Do pineapples belong on pizza?" conversation (and the answer is of course never, fight me). Oftentimes this health status conversation is started by saying something along the lines of, "Oh, are you clean?" That question can mean a variety of things ranging from your household habits to whether you washed your hands recently, but it is not useful language to refer to someone's STI status. Someone's health status is never "clean" or "dirty." Consider language like, "I've tested negative for this (insert test results" or something like, "I tested positive for (insert STI) and am currently on medication to resolve/manage it. Phrases like these remove the value judgement and make for a more comfortable conversation. We need to shift the language to ask "What is your status?" instead of equating a sexually transmitted infection or disease with something dirty.

LET'S TALK ABOUT THE DIFFERENCE BETWEEN AN STI AND STD

An STI is a sexually transmitted infection. An STD is a sexually transmitted disease. With an infection, you're able to clear that up with treatment. An untreated infection can lead to disease though.

With the progress of modern medicine, even the scariest STIs/STDs are no longer a death sentence. Many conditions can be cured or managed with medications. And as always, prevention is half the battle! Knowing your status not only gives you peace of mind when it comes to engaging in sexual activity, but sharing your status with potential partners shows respect for their sexual well-being, as well as your own.

And here's the thing, STIs are very common. Current studies say that one in five people have one. So let's talk about the most common ones.

CURRENT STI FACTS

Chlamydia

According to the CDC, chlamydia is the most frequently reported bacterial STI in the US. There has been a 19% increase since 2014.[42] The bacteria can be transmitted through vaginal, anal, and oral sex. It is curable with antibiotics. Reduce your risk of exposure by using latex condoms.

Gonorrhea

This is caused by the bacterium *Neisseria gonorrhoeae*. Just over

---

42 Centers for Disease Control and Prevention, last modified 2018, https://www.cdc.gov/std/stats18/default.htm.

five hundred eighty thousand people were infected in 2018. This is a 63% increase from 2014.[43] It is transmitted through vaginal, anal, and oral sex. It's curable with antibiotics, and to help reduce your risk, use internal or external latex condoms during vaginal or anal intercourse. While transmission through oral sex is rare, it is still beneficial to use some form of a barrier.

Herpes

Herpes is a very common infection in the US. The most common form is oral herpes, followed by genital herpes, more commonly known as just herpes. The symptoms may come and go, but you will always be a carrier of the virus. It can be acquired through common activities like touching and kissing, but it can also be transmitted sexually via vaginal, anal, and oral sex. And it can be transmitted even if the partner has no symptoms!

Herpes is especially contagious when there are open sores present. To protect yourself from getting herpes, use a condom to limit your risk of exposure. If you have active sores, Planned Parenthood recommends you abstain from any sexual contact until seven days after the sores heal because the virus can be spread to areas that are not protected by a condom. While there is no cure, with medication you can help lessen your outbreak time, and there are also medications to help reduce the number of outbreaks.

It's also important to note that testing for herpes is not usually included in a standard STI panel. You have to ask for that specifically from your healthcare provider. The efficacy

43 Ibid.

of the test can be challenging because you may or may not be exhibiting symptoms of an active infection at the time of testing.

HIV & AIDS

HIV is the abbreviation for the human immunodeficiency virus. It is this virus that causes people to develop AIDS, or acquired immunodeficiency syndrome. The virus can be passed through blood, semen (including pre-ejaculate), breast milk, vaginal fluid, and contaminated needles. Avoid using contaminated needles altogether. And do not engage in intercourse without a condom if there is risk that you or your sexual partner has HIV.

Transmission through oral sex is debated because an open wound or sore is needed to come in contact with the infected fluid. So unless you have a mouth wound or have had dental work recently, technically you are less likely to contract it, but the transmission risk is still there. There may also be increased risk of exposure if you've brushed your teeth or flossed right before oral sex, since that can create microtears in your gums. There is no cure for AIDS yet, but it is not a death sentence like it used to be. With medication, people can still live out full lives while managing their symptoms.

There are also now two treatments, called PrEP and PEP, which can help curb the spread of HIV. PrEP stands for Pre-Exposure Prophylaxis. This can be taken by people who are at risk of contracting HIV. PrEP, when used properly, can stop the spread of HIV through shared needles or unprotected sex. From the CDC, "Studies have shown that PrEP reduces the risk of getting HIV from sex by about 99% when taken consistently. Among people who inject drugs, PrEP reduces the risk of getting HIV by at least 74% when taken consistently."[44]

Conversely, if you do happen to become exposed to HIV, Post-Exposure Prophylaxis, or PEP, is an antiretroviral treatment to help reduce the chance of contracting the virus. It can be taken up to seventy-two hours after the exposure, but sooner is better. According to the CDC, "If you're prescribed PEP, you'll need to take it once or twice daily for 28 days. PEP is effective in preventing HIV when administered correctly, but not 100%."[45]

HPV

HPV stands for human papillomavirus. According to the CDC, this is the most common STI in the US. Some forms of HPV cause genital warts, which are very contagious in their own right. HPV has also been known to cause cervical cancer, but by getting vaccinated against the virus, you can reduce your risk. HPV is transmitted through skin-to-skin contact, so use a condom or a barrier like a dental dam to avoid exposure during oral sex and intercourse.

Syphilis

The bacterium responsible for this STI is *Treponema pallidum*. It is transmitted when there is direct contact to a syphilis sore, and it can infect the external genitalia, anus, rectum, and even your lips and the inside of your mouth! If caught

---

44 Centers for Disease Control and Prevention. Last modified June 4, 2020. https://www.cdc.gov/hiv/basics/prep.html.

45 Centers for Disease Control and Prevention. Last modified August 6, 2019. https://www.cdc.gov/hiv/basics/pep.html.

early enough, within the first year, syphilis can be cured with a single dose of penicillin. There are secondary and tertiary stages of syphilis, which have an increasing risk of medical problems if left untreated. Protect yourself with the use of an internal or external latex condom.

Check your local Planned Parenthood or health department to see if they offer free or low cost STI/HIV testing. Check in your town to find out where clinics are, and then get tested. It's practically painless and you need to know, especially when you're having "the talk" with a new play partner. For those of you who think that having that talk is a mood killer, imagine how bummed out you'd feel if you actually got something—or if you spread an STI to someone else.

Even if a new prospect isn't on the horizon, it's good to know what's going on with you for your own sexual peace of mind. Some STIs can present as asymptomatic in some people, and if left untreated, they can cause damage to your health or fertility. Also, once you know what you have, you can better advise your partners on how to protect themselves in the future.

Be proactive, not reactive. And if you're prescribed antibiotics, ALWAYS remember to take your prescription all the way through! Don't stop half way because you're starting to feel better—you don't want to build up a resistance to the medication and have something like antibiotic-resistant gonorrhea!

WHO SHOULD BE GETTING TESTED?

If you're someone that has had sex, it's probably a good idea to get tested for STIs. This is an encouraged practice if you are beginning a new relationship, you have multiple sex partners, there was nonconsensual nonmonogamy (cheating), or you suspect that you may have an STI. Ignorance is not bliss when considering your sexual health.

Fortunately, many STIs can be cured with medication, and those that cannot be cured can be managed so people can go on to live long, happy, healthy lives. Many times you can find testing services for free or low cost through your local health clinic, and of course your doctor's office. The testing process can be done in one visit, and you should have your results very soon. They will need to do a blood draw finger prick and collect some urine. There is a rapid HIV test, which is a finger prick, and you will know your results within fifteen minutes. While you're there, feel free to ask your healthcare provider any questions—don't be shy. They may ask you questions in turn, like about your sexual partners and what methods of protection you're currently using.

HOW TO HAVE "THE TALK" WITH A NEW PARTNER

Knowing your status is so important. It's one thing to not know your own sexual status if you're not sexually active. But when you decide to play with others, it's your responsibility to know and inform your sexual partners so they can make the best choices for themselves. So, before you engage in any activity, a conversation like this should take place.

Before we go any further, I'd like you to know that I was tested (INSERT WHEN) and my results were (INSERT RESULTS). When was the last time you were tested, and what were your results?

My sexual health matters to me, and I want to make sure we know how best to protect ourselves. When were you tested last, and did you test positive for anything?

Thank you for letting me know you're being treated for chlamydia. I'd feel comfortable if we waited until you finished your medication and were retested before we had sex.

This conversation is best had outside of the bedroom and before you engage in any kind of activity that has a risk of STI transmission. Clearly things like phone sex, video sex, and mutual masturbation don't have the same potential exposure risk as when you're touching each other. Having this conversation in a neutral location gives you both time and perspective to answer freely without feeling the pressure of a clock to answer a certain way just so you can get it on.

And I know that timing can be tricky. It could be date three and the thoughts of sex are shimmering on the periphery of your mind. You don't want to bring it up too soon, but you also don't want to be surprised and have to say, "Shit! We need to talk!" As best you can, gauge the situation and bring it up as soon as you get a whiff that things might be taking an R-rated turn. Even if you had planned for this conversation on date five, and you start kissing on date three, you always have the freedom to stop whatever you're doing and have a conversation with them. Express your concerns, ask questions, and get on the same page so you can get on to whatever you decide to do without wondering "Is this okay?"

BIRTH CONTROL

The discussion you should have about birth control is similar to the conversation above, but here you can discuss specifics on what will work for both of you.

Hey, I'm not trying to catch a baby, so we need to use condoms.

Thanks for letting me know about your herpes diagnosis. It would make me feel comfortable if we used barriers, to be safe about that and as a backup to my birth control pill.

I have an IUD, and because we're going to be fluid bonded, I'm comfortable with just using that as a form of birth control.

These responses can be tailored to your specific boundaries and level of comfort.

CAN I STILL HAVE SEX WITH A PARTNER WITH AN STI?

Yes, but it's up to your discretion. As many STIs are spread through infected bodily fluids, skin-to-skin contact, or contact with mucous membranes, it's important to take steps to reduce the risk of exposure. Using condoms or barriers helps reduce your risk of exposure. There are also many other activities you can engage in with your partner that do not include penetrative sex.

Before you start to explore with real partners in the wild, it's not a bad idea to go over some what-if scenarios and gauge how you would react if a partner disclosed an STI to you. Do your boundaries change if a partner discloses that they have a treatable STI versus a viral infection? Does this change the level of protection/barriers you would want to use? There aren't any right or wrong answers here, just whatever works best for you. Map out what level of risk you're okay with, and if you're presented with that situation in the future, you'll be better prepared to traverse the conversation than if you'd never thought about it in your life.

WHAT TO DO IF A PARTNER HAS HERPES

First of all, good on your partner to let you know they have herpes. With the stigma surrounding STIs/STDs, many people can feel reticent to let people know, even though it's the right thing to do. If we recall, herpes is a virus that cannot be cured, but can be managed through medication.

One out of six people has herpes. But, that being said, not contracting it is a concern I totally understand.

If your partner has an active sore, definitely abstain from any kind of contact. Otherwise, using a barrier method like a condom or dental dam can help protect you from coming into contact with skin that may have viral shedding. The infected skin has to come into contact with you to be transmitted.

Also, research suggests that people who are on suppressive medication (like Valtrex) have an even lower transmission rate to their partner. Some people may have one initial outbreak and then never experience it again. It all just depends on the person.

SAFER SEX AND BIRTH CONTROL

External Condoms

Condoms have been around for the past four hundred years, and their basic intention is still the same: prevent disease and pregnancy. Now, while earlier models were made from things like animal entrails and linen, today's products are made with latex, polyurethane, and some still with animal membranes. Not all condoms are created equal, so try different kinds until you find the one that works for you.

Latex is probably the most popular condom material, and it has amazing elastic properties. Drawbacks to using latex condoms are that some people have latex allergies, and that they are incompatible with oil-based lubricant. The oil will degrade the latex and possibly lead to a breakage. Stick to water-based or silicone lubricants when using latex condoms.

Polyurethane is another type of condom material. It is thinner than latex and can conduct body heat better, giving the wearer a more "natural" feel. All lubricants, including oil-based ones, can be used with this type of condom.

Animal membrane condoms are commonly known as "lambskin" condoms. The name is a misnomer because the condoms are actually made from sheep's intestines. Unlike latex and polyurethane condoms, animal membrane condoms do not protect against most STD/STIs, including HIV. Because this is a natural material, there are holes in the membranes that are large enough to allow in viruses, but small enough to stop sperm, which are larger.

Condoms can also come in different varieties of textures, colors, and flavors. Some may be studded or ribbed to add additional external pleasure to the receiver. Some are flavored, which can be beneficial when having oral sex because many find the taste of unflavored condoms unpalatable (although flavored condoms shouldn't be used for vaginal sex, as they can contain sugars that may upset the pH balance of the vagina, potentially causing yeast infections). Some may be colored, or even glow in the dark. They also come in different sizes.

A few words of caution when using external condoms:

- Don't keep condoms in your wallet. The constant pressure, rubbing, and friction can compromise the condom and lead to breakage.
- Don't open it with your teeth! You risk tearing or poking a hole in the condom. Open it with your hands and save the teeth for elsewhere.
- Only put a condom on an erect penis.
- Use a new condom for every act of intercourse. If you're doing anal sex and want to switch to vaginal sex or oral sex, grab a new one.
- Keep condoms at room temperature. Extreme temperatures can also compromise the condom's integrity.
- After ejaculation and before the penis goes soft, hold the base of the condom and carefully pull out of your partner, ensuring that no semen spills out.

Internal Condoms

Internal condoms can be used for both anal and vaginal sex. With external condoms, you need a hard penis to put them on, but with internal condoms, you can insert the condom and be ready to go ahead of time (up to eight hours!). Similar rules apply to the storage and application of an internal condom.

▸ No wallet storage.

▸ No opening with teeth.

▸ These usually come prelubricated, but have lube on hand just in case.

▸ Internal condoms have two soft "rings" in them—a smaller ring that is meant to be inserted, and a larger ring that is meant to remain outside the body. Relax and slowly insert the smaller ring into the vagina. Pinch it so it's like an oval for easier insertion. You want that to sit at the back end of the vagina, resting against the cervix.

▸ For anal sex, same moves apply. Pinch and insert. Some people recommend removing the inner ring for anal sex, but messing around with it could lead to inadvertent tears. Just leave it be.

▸ Once it's inserted, fully open the larger ring over the vulva or anus to act as a bullseye for your penis or toy.

▸ Guide your partner into the larger ring. Make sure they don't slip to the side and penetrate you outside of the condom.

▸ Once you're finished, twist the outer ring and remove the condom. Put it in the trash.

Dental Dam/Glove Hack

Dental dams are great if you want to protect yourself from exposure from tissues or fluids, particularly during oral sex. They prevent your mouth from coming into direct contact with your partner's skin, but they're thin enough for you to still be able to feel the warmth of their skin. Best used if you keep one side dedicated to your mouth and the other to your partner's parts.

If you find yourself without access to a dental dam, it's easy to DIY your own from a condom. Unroll the condom and cut the tip off. Make a vertical slit up the side, and you've crafted your own dental dam. You can also use a glove to make a dental dam with a built-in hole explorer. Cut all of the finger parts off of the glove, only leaving the thumb part attached. Cut vertically up the pinky side of the glove, and you've made yourself a dental dam with a place for a finger or a tongue to fit into.

As with external condoms, make sure you're not reusing dental dams and not flushing them down the toilet.

The Pill

This is a medication taken daily to prevent pregnancy. They come with varying levels of hormones, which can thicken the mucus in your cervix (so as to make the passage of sperm into your uterus very difficult), halt ovulation (no egg, no pregnancy), or thin your endometrium (which can prevent the egg from taking up residence there). It does not prevent the transmission of STIs.

The IUD

This is an intrauterine device. It is a small *T*-shaped device that has to be inserted by a medical professional. There are hormonal and nonhormonal options on the market. The hormone-containing ones do the same things that the pill does: thicken the cervical mucus and make it difficult for sperm to travel up. The nonhormonal copper IUD works by stopping sperm from meeting an egg.

My IUD Story

In 2012, I decided to get an IUD, or intrauterine device. This was after a long process of weighing the pros and cons for this type of birth control. According to Planned Parenthood, "There are 5 different brands of IUDs that are FDA approved for use in the United States: Paragard, Mirena, Kyleena, Liletta, and Skyla."[46] I chose Paragard. It was the most appealing because it was hormone-free, lasted up to ten years, and was one of the most economical forms of birth control out there.

I had to wait until I was on my period because that would be when my cervix would be most receptive to receiving the IUD. May 17th was the fateful day that I popped 600 mg of ibuprofen (they recommend that you take some pain relievers about thirty minutes before you come in) and drove myself to the clinic.

What I really enjoy about my gynecological clinic is that there are no harsh, glaring fluorescent lights starring you back in the face as you lie on the table wearing that gown with too many holes in it. The room is tastefully painted and has a little lamp emitting a nice friendly glow. I was relaxed and going over what I knew about the contraception and the insertion procedure (thanks YouTube!).

Finally, my midwife and her nurse came into the room. I found out that this procedure was one of my midwife's favorite things to do! She asked me if I had any questions about the copper IUD and I said no, telling her that I'm a sexologist, so I'm pretty familiar with the product. She warmed up the speculum, lubed it up, and we were off.

---

46 Planned Parenthood, last modified 2020, https://www.plannedparenthood.org/learn/birth-control/iud.

My midwife talked about each step of the procedure before she did it, and I was following along in my head. She explained to me that because I'd never had a child, my cervix had never been opened and that she may have a little difficulty getting it in, but she had never failed at an implantation, so no worries.

She sounded my uterus (measured it with a sound, which is a smooth cylindrical metal instrument), through my cervix, to see how deep she needed to insert the IUD.

"You're going to feel some pressure."

Not so bad.

She opened the package containing the IUD, and I was shown how the arms were folded down in the insertion device along with the little copper coils. She warned that I may feel a little more pressure than before and that I should take a breath. On the count of three . . .

One . . .

Two . . .

Three . . .

In.

Fuck.

Hello cramp from hell! I tensed up immediately and was shocked at how much it hurt. I didn't think it would be much worse than the sound going through my cervix, but it was.

After breaking out in a cold sweat, I was still trying to keep it cool. She said that I would probably have some intense cramping the first few days and an extended period/spotting. After six to eight days the cramping should subside, and I should be back to normal. I listened as she told me that she cut the strings about 3 cm so that I could check them, and that they would eventually soften with time. She said I did great and told me that I would be good and pregnancy free until 2022. AMAZING, but I was too uncomfortable to make any more small talk.

I got dressed and walked to the desk to sign out and do the paperwork stuff and schedule my six-week check. All the while, I could feel my uterus contracting more and more as time went on. She was not very happy with me, my uterus. I scrambled to my car, just wanting to get home to my bed and painkillers. I have never been more thankful that I live only a mile away from my clinic, but it seemed like the longest mile! I was sitting in my car, audibly breathing and telling myself to relax . . . relax . . . maybe it's all in your head . . . get a grip Meg! As soon as I got home, I ran upstairs and curled into the fetal position.

I am a worst-case scenario planner, and all I could think about was "What if something went wrong?" "What if they have to take it out and put another in?" and other crazy things like that. I don't ever recall reading anything online about the crazy intense cramping that the insertion may cause, which is part of the reason why I'm sharing this. Contraction after contraction. I could not believe how uncomfortable it was.

Fast forward a few days, and my period ended, but I still had wicked awful cramps. The cramps weren't the ordinary menstrual cramps that I was used to, but "It feels like I'm going into labor" cramps. I completely went over the six to eight additional days of cramping. Some days they were debilitating. I took a lot of ibuprofen and Vicodin in those two weeks. But one day, the pain was gone! It was such a relief.

I'm at the point now that I actually forget that I have it

in me. I'm very happy now with this birth control. It wasn't my intention to scare or dissuade you from getting an IUD with this story. (In fact, a friend told me that some clinics now give their patients drugs before inserting the IUD.) I wanted to share my story so that you could have a first-hand account of my journey, and so you would understand the side effects you might have. Would I go through this again? Absolutely. Having a couple weeks of cramps is a more than acceptable price to pay for ten years of nonhormonal protection against pregnancy. Also, it is one of the most economical birth control options around, at about $6.25[47] a month. Win-win.

I still recommend that you use an additional barrier method of contraception because, while an IUD protects against pregnancy, it does not protect against STD/STIs.

Fertility Awareness Method

This method is done by tracking your ovulation. It's also known as the rhythm method. There are many different apps and devices you can use to track your ovulation. Many of them rely on your BBT, or basal body temperature. You will see a slight spike in temperature as your body gets ready to ovulate. You can also track where you're at in your cycle by checking your cervical mucus. This method requires consistent practice so that you know when you're leading up to those fertile days. You can choose to couple this with another form of birth control as well.

---

47 This number is based on the cost of my IUD—costs may vary.

UNPROTECTED SEX

Oops, that wasn't part of the plan. Unprotected sex happens and its totally okay, so don't freak out! Forgive yourself for being human. Try to do better next time. There are probably a whole host of feelings going through your mind, but focus on what you can control right now.

If you haven't yet discussed your status with your partner, now is the time. People, especially penis owners, can present as asymptomatic for STIs. You can't look at a person and know with any certainty if they do or do not have an STI. Why take a risk with something as important as your sexual health? Being sexually active and responsible go hand in hand, so please get tested!

If you think you have been exposed to the human immunodeficiency virus (HIV), talk to your healthcare provider about the benefits of taking post exposure prophylaxis, or PEP. As we discussed earlier, in research it's been suggested that this can help lower your risk of HIV infection after unintentional exposure.

If you're someone who can get pregnant, consider using emergency contraception (EC). It's best to take it as soon as possible (do you know where you are in your cycle?), but EC can be used up to seventy-two hours after unprotected sex (89% effective).[48] It works by preventing fertilization or implantation in the uterus. Skip the expensive pregnancy tests. It's too soon to know anything beyond "Oops, I just had unprotected sex."

As they say, "No Ls, just lessons." I'm sure this experience

---

48 Plan B One-Step, last modified 2020, https://www.planbonestep.com/faqs/.

will stick with you for a while, and that's a good thing. Like that time when you eagerly scooped up some hot soup and burned your tongue—in the future, you won't forget to let it cool off first. Do the work of testing beforehand so you can be ready when the time comes and prevent a situation like this from happening in the future. Your sexual health is your responsibility, so treat it with respect for the sake of yourself and others.

CHAPTER 9:
EMPOWERED SEX WITH NEAR STRANGERS

Even if a long-term relationship isn't on your radar, you can absolutely still have fulfilling sex with near strangers that can meet your needs. All you need is a willing subject, some communication, and maybe a pre-made sexy checklist of things you can do together. I'm sure you've had enough awkward sex, so here are some tips to leave that behind and make your early relationship encounters the best they can be.

YES/NO/MAYBE LIST

As we all know, no partner is a mind reader. Unless you're clairvoyant, then disregard the following. For the rest of us muggles, we need to have conversations with our partners. Sometimes, in new pairings especially, it can seem like the right time never prevents itself to bring up our sexual wish list. But, you're in luck! A yes/no/maybe list may be just what you need to spark a conversation and secretly glean if your partner is as freaky as you.

A yes/no/maybe list is a compilation of many sexual acts

ranging from mild to wild. Think of it as an ungraded quiz for your sexual likes and dislikes. If you're totally into something, you'd select yes. If you're curious or have had some interest in something, you'd select maybe. And if something is a hard pass, you'd select no.

For maximum effectiveness, take this quiz alone and give a copy to your partner to take too. Then, once finished, join up and go over your results. Imagine a sexy Venn diagram in your mind, where you find overlapping things that you and your partner both enjoy! Taking the assessment separately gives you the freedom to respond your own way without the pressure of a partner next to you waiting for you to check the "yes" box next to shrimping (which is sucking on toes BTW).

Analingus
Anal play
Bondage
Blindfolds
CBT
Cock rings
Cuckholding
Cunnilingus
Cumshots
Cyber Sex
Dirty Talk
Domination & submission
Erotic Massage
Exhibitionism
Felching
Fellatio
Figging
Fingering
Fisting

Gags
Golden showers
Group sex
Hot wifing
Intercourse
Masturbation
Multiple penetration
Nipple play
Needle play
Pearl necklaces
Pegging
Phone sex
Prostate play
Quickies
Rainbow showers
Role play
Rough play
Scissoring
Sensory deprivation
Sex clubs

Sex parties
Sexting
Shibari
Shrimping
S&M
Sploshing
Spanking/impact play
Strip tease
Threesomes
Vacuum pumps
Vibrators
Voyeurism
Watching porn
Water sports
Wax play

NONBORING WAYS TO ASK FOR CONSENT

Consent is required any time you engage in sexual activity with someone. It needs to be freely given and it can be revoked at any time. Just because you agreed to do something once does not mean that you want to do that same thing again.

Naysayers think that asking for consent can ruin the mood, but I say consent is only boring if you are. Consider these two conversation starters:

Can I kiss your lips while squeezing your breast every three seconds?

That's very weird, so yeah that might ruin the mood for some. Consider this alternative:

If I were to kiss you right now, I'd start by exploring your beautiful lips with my mouth. I want to know what you taste like. And while I'm doing that, I want to massage your soft breasts, feel your nipples grow hard under my touch.

Don't mind me, I'm just fanning myself over here. That second one was way hotter and got the same points across.

If you're still feeling at a loss for how to start the conversation, try some of these phrases:

What do you want to do?
Can I touch you here?
What would turn you on?
Do you want more?
Are you horny?
Do you want me to stop?

How about we try . . .
What sounds like fun?
Is this good?
You want more?

CONDOM USE DURING A ONE-NIGHT STAND

I think the best way to bring up condom use during a one-night stand is before you get into the bedroom. An easy entrance into the safer-sex conversation can be something simple like, "What does safer sex mean to you?" That way you can see what your partner is thinking and see if that aligns with what you're comfortable with.

I know what you're thinking: at what point during the one-night stand do you suggest the conversation be brought up? Pre-foreplay? During foreplay?

I definitely recommend having the condom conversation before any touching happens. Run through a list of things you're into and things you aren't into with your partner before you start to engage in any sexual activity. Once you have the knowledge of your partner's dos and don'ts, the entire experience will run much more smoothly—and that includes asking for condom use.

WHAT IF MY PARTNER DOESN'T WANT TO WEAR A CONDOM?

If your partner is against using a condom, I would definitely inquire why that is. Whatever reason they give, valid or not, is their decision. But when it comes to having sex with you, if condoms are nonnegotiable, say so. If you were planning to use a condom as your form of birth control and STI protection, make that clear, and don't engage in any activities that feel risky. That may just mean you don't have penetrative sex that night. There are many other activities you can do that do not require penetration and condom use, but whatever you do, don't feel pressured into compromising your values.

BE CONFIDENT

Have you ever heard the saying "Life is about the journey, not the destination?" Your sensual journey should operate under the same belief system. Pressure from society, our partners, or ourselves can manifest itself in many different ways, but most often, we get caught up worrying about the small stuff. You may catch yourself thinking, "Does he see that spot I missed shaving? Please don't look at my armpits!" or "Ugh! I should have stuck with that thirty-day squat challenge!"

Stressing out over these types of things can bog us down mentally and make it difficult to enjoy the experience. More often than not, your partner does not notice whatever you're worrying about, but they may pick up on your physical cues that something is off. Just relax and keep it simple.

If you ever have to fake anything in the bedroom, fake confidence! Give real-time feedback to your partner or better yet, show them exactly what you desire. Remember that nerves are normal and everyone gets them, even people who seem confident. Go after what you want and if something should go awry, so be it! You're allowed to laugh. Remember that intimacy with your partner is supposed to be fun.

TRY SOMETHING NEW

New partner, new activity! Try something new with your partner and discover more about them in the process. You'll likely have things in common, but they may have some hobbies or pastimes you've never experienced before. Being open to their suggestions can be exciting and can help strengthen your bond, unless it's tandem kayaking and you flip the boat. I heard that from a friend, I swear. And new partners may have exciting, previously unexplored activities for the bedroom as well. Use this opportunity to try positions or toys you've never tried before. Even if you don't excel at your new activity, it's sure to make for fun memories!

HOW TO TALK ABOUT YOUR BODY

Sometimes we know what we want to say in our mind, but it becomes challenging when we actually have to articulate it. Factors like anxiety and judgment can make us feel like our concerns aren't valid, or that they don't need to be voiced. Especially when it comes to sexual relationships with others, you need to feel comfortable using your voice.

Painful Sex

In an informal study on the prevalence of painful sex done by the team at OhNut—a device you can wear to minimize pain during sex by reducing the depth of penetration—they found that there were many great reasons why people tell their partners when sex is painful. When asked why they speak up, 25% of their respondents said they wanted to make sure that both parties felt good during sex. Other responses included "they wouldn't want to hurt me," "communication is key," and "pain outweighs pleasure."[49] With those facts in hand,

---

49 "5 Ways to Tell Your Partner Is Uncomfortable—During Sex," OhNut. last modified February 4, 2020, https://ohnut.co/blogs/journal/5-ways-to-tell-your-partner-sex-is-uncomfortable-during-sex.

how do you convey to your partner that you're experiencing pain? I think that verbal communication is the best way to get your message across to your partner. If you're experiencing pain during any sexual activity, try saying something like:

Oh, hold on a minute.
Can we slow down for a second?
Can we try a different position?
Will you touch me here instead?

These sentences don't have to "kill the mood," but they still convey that a change needs to take place. Ideally your partner will respond positively to your request, and you can go on with your bad self.

Body Issues/Injury/Disability

If you have an injury or disability, or any health issue that is vital for your partner to know about, you need to tell them. They don't know what they don't know. You can try conversation starters very matter of factly.

I have an injury from a car accident, so I can't be violently jostled around. I can't have any rough sex or hands around my neck.

Hold on—I think I need some lube!

Can you grab a pillow because I need extra support under my back? Thanks!

It's as easy and as difficult as that. Having a partner who you trust, who respects you, and who is a good communicator is important to this process.

If you have a disability or are experiencing a prolonged medical issue that isn't going to go away with a few positive affirmations, communication is key (again!). Talk to your partner about where your comfort level is regarding certain activities. Maybe you don't have the energy/ability to do [_____], but you can always cuddle, kiss, or something along those lines. Being able to express your boundaries is important, especially when considering a new partner. You can use the following lines to help broach this subject.

> *Hey, I just wanted to let you know that after my treatment, I don't have enough energy to do [_____].*
> *Right now I'm having a high pain day. Can we do [_____] instead?*
> *I'm just not physically up for [_____] right now. Thank you for understanding.*

There is absolutely nothing wrong with having needs or boundaries, and expressing them. It is encouraged, and any partner with their salt will respect that.

HOW TO ASK FOR WHAT YOU WANT

An easy way to get what you want is to ask for what you want. Start these conversations off as early as you can in your relationship. This can be done by sharing your fantasies with someone, or by sharing your Yes/No/Maybe list with your partner (see previous section on the Yes/No/Maybe list).

When giving feedback directly related to the sex you've

been having, remember that your partner is human too, and sometimes they might experience hurt feelings. Try to have a positive approach when you're going to talk about something that isn't working well. The "positive sandwich" approach can be helpful in the right situation:

I love when you fuck me from behind. I'd like it if you didn't pull my hair while you did it. I like being able to look back and see your face.

You slide the change request between the two positives, and it lessens the blow. Sounds much nicer than just, "Don't pull my hair when you're fucking me from behind."

You can also have this conversation during your post-play debrief as you make plans for your future encounters.

Next time, I'd love to be on top and use a toy. How does that sound to you?

I liked that we tried reverse cowgirl, but it wasn't for me. Can we stick to doggy style and missionary?

If ever you want to try something new, consider using the old standby of, "Hey, I read an article that mentioned (insert activity). Would you ever be interested in trying something like that?" It takes the pressure off your partner and allows them to say no to the article and not to you. If they say yes, mission accomplished! If they say no, you never have to bring up sploshing again! Sneaky.

HOW TO SAY NO

Saying no seems simple enough, but when we add the layer of another person during sex, it can seem like a more daunting task. By all means, you have the right to say no in any form, at any time, but sometimes you'd like to make it a "not right now." Either way, here are some ways to say no:

> *I'm really interested in getting to know you better first.*
> *I'm not ready to do (insert whatever).*
> *Oh, I'm not into that.*
> *No.*

Make sure that the person you're with is hearing you. Be clear and direct with your delivery. Also, do not let them pressure you into something that you're not ready to do. A yes under coercion is not a freely given yes. Do not let beatdown tactics make you compromise your boundaries.

If you've already started to engage in activities, you can still say no at any point.

> *Hey, I've changed my mind. I'm not ready for (insert whatever).*

They might have questions for you, and you can give them an explanation, but you don't owe them anything. Ideally you're with someone who respects you and is willing to meet you at your boundaries.

CHAPTER 10:
TIPS FOR GREAT SEX

---

know we've been on this journey together to embolden you to own your sexuality while single, which may mean more solo play, but there may come a time when you want to have "plays well with others" included on your dating resume. We already know that we don't *need* to seek out others to have fulfilling, deliciously orgasmic, mind-blowing sex (see masturbation chapter), but sometimes we may have to consider someone else in the equation. Whether this is your first or fortieth time having sex with someone new, there are always some constant variables to consider. It's just like riding a bike, if you used to have sex with your bike.

As I've said, when it comes to sex with others, communication is crucial. In addition to having consent, it's foundational to any kind of relationship. I like to say that if you aren't able to talk about what you want to do sexually with your partner, you shouldn't be doing those things sexually with your partner.

This isn't a movie, where we're kissing for two minutes

and then suddenly we're in penetration mode with moaning and orgasm shortly thereafter. Real life doesn't work like that. You should hopefully have enough comfort with your partner, even a brand new partner, to speak up and talk about any concerns you have sexually, ESPECIALLY if they involve pain! Unless that is part of the play you're seeking, your partner shouldn't want to be causing you pain.

Whenever there needs to be communication about a sensitive subject, I always recommend having this outside of the bedroom at a neutral location. Having this conversation during the throes of sex can skew answers and/or make a partner feel pressured to answer a certain way. You want your partner to be actively listening and willing to work with you on ways to make sex more comfortable. They should also be understanding that sometimes sex may be halted, even if it's mid-act, in case of any sort of discomfort or for any other reason: Consent 101.

IMPORTANCE OF INTIMACY

Intimacy helps strengthen the bond in a relationship. It allows you to be honest with your partner without the fear of judgment about something you say or ask for. It definitely isn't required for a positive sexual encounter, though. It's an added layer to help fortify the trust, and can also add an element of vulnerability to your encounters.

Intimacy can make people uncomfortable because it asks them to be vulnerable. You're opening yourself up, and you have to trust that the person you're with will receive what you've shared well and not abuse you with that closeness. People are afraid of judgment, so the safer route is to not rock the boat and just go along to get along, even if that means not speaking up for what you truly want. But that route often makes for less satisfying sex and relationships.

You can help create a sense of comfort around intimacy by starting with small acts of intimacy. Holding hands is a great start. Tell each other your fears or worries. Write a note. These small acts can be a great way to start to build intimacy. As you grow more comfortable with the different acts, you can move on to larger displays.

KISSING

Maybe you're a little out of practice, or you're practicing to pucker up for the first time. Kissing doesn't have to be anything that intimidates you. There are so many different ways to kiss, but the two main techniques are either lips closed or lips open. While engaging in either, keep these factors in mind.

Fresh Breath

I'm not discounting the cute morning breath kiss, because that has its own place in the world. But freshness is key, especially for a new kiss with someone. Don't overlook the benefits that brushing and flossing your teeth can provide. Bad breath comes from old food particles starting to decay in your mouth. That does not sound or smell appetizing at all. If you're coming from a dinner, pop in a mint or some gum.

Soft Lips

This is where that lip balm comes in handy! It's pleasant to kiss soft lips, so consider keeping them lush and plump. If in a pinch, you can moisten your lips with your tongue pre-kiss. Don't go in tongue first! Start with light kisses that just barely brush your partner's lips. Once things have progressed, feel free to increase the intensity of your kiss. Pretend you're licking an ice cream cone for a guide to the right pace—slowly and sensuously.

Eyes Open/Eyes Closed

This is really up to you. For me, I think it's great to go in with eyes closed and take a peek at your partner if you want. It might be a little jarring to go in with eyes wide open. It's up to you though.

Head Tilt

Because of the way our heads are shaped, we need to tilt our heads to achieve a good kissing position. This allows you to have airflow to your nose and keeps you from smashing faces. Also be mindful that you don't smash teeth or connect your braces together like in middle school.

Don't Forget about Your Body

While you can both be just touching lips, with your butts out, consider stepping into each other and embracing. Use your hands to circle your partner's waist or rub their back. You can run them up the neck of your partner and fist your hands into their hair, or just press them close against you. There are so many possibilities.

Benefits of Kissing

Kisses don't have to be boring by any means. Switch it up and kiss other erogenous zones, like their ears and neck. Watch your partner's body cues and go with the flow. Use a combination of the above techniques to make your next kiss unforgettable.

Kissing comes with many health benefits too:

- Over thirty facial muscles are involved in making a kiss happen. Using these muscles can help keep your cheeks tight and in perfect pucker shape.
- Looking to burn some calories? While kissing, you can burn up to three calories per minute. I know it's menial, but it is still a win-win.
- Stressed out? Try kissing. Oxytocin, otherwise known as the love hormone, is released when you kiss and can help in calming you down. It can also reaffirm your romantic attachment to your partner.

HAVE A SENSE OF HUMOR

All of that said, sometimes even the best of us have sexual bloopers. If you can't laugh during sex, you're doing it wrong. I knew all of these stories would finally come in handy!

Christening Anecdote

Something that had seemed so promising took a turn that no one could have anticipated.

This guy and I were co-workers, and after about a week of serious sexting, we both knew it was time to nut up or shut up. He invited me over to his house and it was on.

As soon as I walked in the door, our mouths were on each other. We stumbled into his bedroom and clothes went flying. He was an amazing kisser. His mouth laid a trail of kisses, licks, and bites between my breasts, down my stomach, and finally between my legs.

He was merciless. His tongue seemed to be everywhere all at once. He was turning me on and taking me so high, I knew it was only going to be a matter of minutes before he drove me to orgasm. My breath was coming in gasps, my legs were shaking, and I was beginning to moan.

It was happening, I was coming. Oh my god was I coming. At that point I was moaning uncontrollably, but that didn't mean he stopped with his tongue assault. Just when I thought it couldn't get any hotter, any more intense, any more exciting, it did.

That's when he sneezed on me.

Yup . . . awesome. Imagine someone taking a spray bottle, like you'd use for an orchid, and finely misting your vulva, but instead of water, it's a cold shot of dissipated mucous particles.

My moans were immediately replaced with laughter. I could not believe that had just happened. I know you should celebrate when a new "ship" launches, but he didn't have to christen the boat. I was laughing so hard I started to tear up. Looking back, I think that this guy may have taken an ego hit, but come on, you just straight up sneezed on my crotch.

Needless to say, I forgave him. (It was great oral, and that's a hard skill to find these days). But let it be known to all, if you feel a sneeze coming on, please turn your head.

Liquor Dick Anecdote

It was a late night after heavy alcohol consumption at the bar, and I was heading home with my squeeze of the month. We got back to his place and promptly hopped into bed. We made out for a bit, and then he began to give me oral. It was fantastic. (No really, I mean it. It wasn't the alcohol talking.)

We went back to making out for a while, and I wanted to return the favor.

I slowly slid my body down his torso, being oh so sexy, and nestled nicely between his legs. And for the record, I think I have quite prodigious oral sex skills, so this was going to be no trouble at all to get him off and then get both of us to sleep.

Cue liquor dick.

Liquor dick is the phenomenon where a man has erectile dysfunction as a result of too much alcohol consumption. Also known as whiskey dick.

I didn't let that stop me. I was pulling out all of my best moves, and oh he was loving it, but he was nowhere near finishing. By now, not only was I tired from all of the dancing and boozing that happened prior to this, but my mouth was getting tired too. But I'm no quitter, so I kept going.

It took so long, I was almost to the point of falling asleep with his dick in my mouth.

. . . Oh wait, that did happen.

The next thing I remember, he was gently shaking me saying, "Hey, did you fall asleep?"

Umm yup. There I was, my head laid on his inner thigh with his dick in my mouth.

Fail.

Happy Hour Anecdote

I was out to brunch with my best friend Jennie, and I always like to share my escapades with her because something out of the ordinary always happens. That day stands out in my memory not because of the sex story, but what happened after it.

I was dating an older guy we will call "Neighborhood Dad." We would have late-night hookups frequently. One night he called me to come over, and I said sure, I'll be over shortly. He had shared custody of his daughters, so we didn't see each other with great regularity. Now that it had been a while since I'd seen Neighborhood Dad, I'd stopped shaving. I thought, hmm, can I speed shave and then make it over there in a timely manner? Let's find out!

Jennie and I were leaving the restaurant when I was telling this story. We both had to go to the bathroom, so I just kept talking. The bathroom had two stalls, one for each of us. The story continues.

I told her all about how Neighborhood Dad went down on me. How he expertly used his fingers and said nasty things. To be fair, I couldn't really hear her well. I thought she might have been making encouraging sounds or laughing to let me know she was tracking the story.

I told her that after I came, Neighborhood Dad lifted his head from between my legs and smiled up at me. WITH A LONG PUBIC HAIR ON ONE OF HIS TEETH. By now I'm laughing, because how absurd is that? That is shit you see in a movie. Jennie is most definitely laughing now. We both exit the stalls at the same time, and there is another woman in the bathroom laughing along with us.

It takes a lot for me to get hot in the cheeks. This was one of those moments. Jennie had tears streaming down her face, and said she tried to tell me that someone else had walked into the bathroom. I don't know how hard she tried though.

I of course apologized to the woman, and she laughed it off saying it was cool.

And if you're wondering if I told Neighborhood Dad about the errant hair. Nope!

TIPS FOR PLAY WITH A NEW PARTNER

First of all, no two bodies are the same. Even if you think you've had every kind of sex out there, you haven't had it with this particular person, so plan accordingly with these tips.

Anxiety

Didn't think I was going to lead off with this one, did you? Feeling anxious is totally normal when it comes to new partner experiences. Anxiety can be helped by simply talking to your partner about your fears, concerns, whatever. Whether that means easing into being sexual with each other or disclosing some health issues, you deserve the right to speak up about whatever is weighing heavy on you. Do not be afraid to reach out to a therapist for help if this is something that continues to distress you.

Check-Ins

Ask yourself how you're feeling. What are your senses telling you? Do you feel safe? What is your mental state? Some nerves are okay, but if fear has you hitting the brakes and slowing things down, try to figure out why.

Be Confident in Your Body

Listen, once the clothes come off, the last thing on your partner's mind is going to be that random nipple hair that came out of nowhere. If you don't make a big deal of it, they won't either. Only when you draw attention to something do partners ever see our self-perceived flaws.

Remember our body map exercise from Chapter 4, and how we worked on building up our body confidence? Share your body map with your partner. Show them how you like to be touched. Don't be afraid to ask for what you want.

MY PARTNER IS HOTTER THAN ME

First, we should always consider that "hotness" is in the eye of the beholder. Second, when you see someone you consider hot, try not to make it a reductive thing, like "Oh you're so hot you must not be interested in me." We humans are complex, multifaceted creatures. But with that being said, if you're feeling uneasy with your hot partner, talk to them about it. Don't say, "You're too hot and it makes me insecure." But delve deeper and ask yourself where your insecurity comes from.

Are you worried about the attention they may receive? Do you think they have eyes for the next best thing (not you)? Is it setting off your insecurities about your own body? Try to pinpoint where it's coming up for you, and then discuss with your partner. They can hopefully allay some of your worries, but ultimately it's your own work to do, not theirs. They can't change who they are.

Conversely, yes, dating someone hot can be a self-esteem boost, but not in a gross trophy sense.

Again, don't be reductive. Yes, it's awesome your partner is hot, but what else is special about them that you like? Be proud of all that they are, not just how many people break their neck trying to get a second look as they walk by.

Honestly, unless you're a mind reader, you don't know what someone is looking for. So if you see someone you're attracted to, just put your best foot forward and say hey. You may be surprised. But remember, too, people have the right to say no, and it's your job to respect that and not take it personally. Remember, there are many reasons why someone may not be interested.

HOW TO HAVE A HOT ONE-NIGHT STAND

If you want to have a one-night stand, make sure you're doing it for the right reasons—that this is something you 100% want to do, and you aren't being pressured or under the impression that this will make someone like you more.

Dress Up

This is the perfect excuse to wear that hot little number you've been wearing dancing. Wear something that makes you feel confident. You're planning on showing someone the goods, so make the goods look their best in whatever outfit you love.

Be Selfish

It's not as bad as it sounds. Speak up in bed! Ask for what you want. What kind of touch? What kind of pressure, speed, intensity? Where do you want them to pleasure you? Make sure you are an active and satisfied participant. Your pleasure is just as important as theirs.

Laugh

Another key component of a good one-night stand is being willing to let yourself laugh. Slip-ups or mistakes can happen, and laughter is an easy way to break the tension. Especially since this is a new partner and you don't know their body well. Have a good sense of humor and have fun.

TURNING A ONE-NIGHT STAND INTO A RELATION-SHIP

Sometimes, you can turn a hookup into a dating relationship. This conversation is best had outside of the bedroom and not directly after you've just had sex. You might not get a fully honest answer from them right after sex. They may be reticent to answer while you're both lying there naked.

If this was a one-night stand with someone you'll continue to speak to, whenever you next talk, mention that you'd like to do something together. This isn't the time to say "Last night was great, let's do it again," unless you're strictly referring to the sex. Mention a specific activity and gauge their interest.

If you've been solely hooking up with someone for a while and you want to make a transition, this should be an in-person conversation. Again, not in bed. You can say that you've really enjoyed hooking up with them AND spending time with them. Are they feeling the same?

You have to prepare yourself for rejection because that is always a possibility. It takes two to be in a relationship, so if they're only feeling the hookup, that's okay—a good hookup is a good hookup. If you're still feeling like you want something more, you owe it to both of you to speak up and say something. If there isn't clear communication and you continue doing what you're doing without speaking up, resentments can form, and that isn't beneficial to any relationship.

ONE-NIGHT STAND ANECDOTE

I met this guy where most romances begin: a dating app. After talking on the app for a while, we decided to meet up for drinks. This was summer, so we decided to opt for a rooftop bar. We ordered some food and split a bottle of wine. I cannot tell you where the hours went because at one point it was 6:30 and then our server was telling us that it's the last call and they're getting ready to close. There was something magnetic about this guy. Everything just clicked and flowed—it was like you imagine a perfect date to be.

We didn't want the night to end, so we decided to take a walk by the river. If you know Grand Rapids, the walk along the Grand River downtown can be very quaint. We strolled hand in hand past the antique carousel in the public museum, looked at the lush gardens, and had the bright lights of the city as our backdrop. We ended up walking on the blue pedestrian bridge that spans the distance of the river. We stopped in the middle of the bridge and just looked out over the water. I know some of you may be gagging or eye-rolling, but I swear this is what happened next. He turned me around and gave me one of those leading men, violins-swelling kisses that you see in movies. It was too perfect. As cliché as it sounds, I said, "I don't want this date to end." He said that he didn't either.

This is where the story becomes a bit ill advised. I said, "Are you up for something crazy?" He replied yes. I suggested that we drive to the lakeshore. I didn't know if this guy was an ax murderer. I was young, and wild, and free. We parked in a neighborhood and walked hand in hand over the dunes with only moonlight as our guide. The woods opened up to an empty beach with grass gently waving in the breeze. As any Michigan Mermaid does, I stripped off my dress and bra and ran into the waves. He soon followed after me, and we connected in the water. As an aside, if you have not had the privilege of being naked in water (no, the shower and tub do not count), you should really try it.

The cool lake water on our skin was magical. It was a full moon with light cloud cover. A gorgeous night. He lifted me up from the water and had me floating on my back while he went down on me. ARE YOU KIDDING ME?! It was too perfect. I came, and of course I saw stars. We made our way back to the beach where he laid a towel down, pulled out a condom (so responsible!), and we had sex on the beach. It is, still to this day, one of the hottest one-night stands I have ever had.

MORNING-AFTER ETIQUETTE

So you just hooked up with someone—now what? If it's still nighttime, there is nothing wrong with engaging in little afterglow chat and then getting your clothes and heading out. It's a little rude if you suddenly pop up right after sex and run for the door.

If you end up spending the night at their house, there are a lot of possibilities that can happen. By all means, you're welcome to get up in the morning, start putting your clothes on, and head for the door. They may wake up (or were they awake the whole time and just pretending to be asleep?) and ask what's the rush. This is a cue that you're welcome to stay, or maybe that they want to have coffee with you. Maybe they want some morning sex. If they wake up and don't make any efforts to ask you to stay, that's a sign to go ahead and leave.

If they spend the night at your place, similar scenario. If you want things to continue, and you want to have breakfast together, offer that option to them. If you'd like them to get a move on, you can mention that you have an appointment to get to.

Either way, it can be a fluid situation, and the better you communicate about it, the less awkward it will be. And BTW, that morning sojourn home, wearing last night's clothes, is no longer called the walk of shame. We've rebranded it and are now calling it the stride of pride. High five on gettin' some!

BEDROOM ESSENTIALS

Want to make sure your bedroom is equipped with all of the essentials to make for a great night of sexual play? Make your list and be sure to include these items.

Lube

It is super essential. Have you ever heard the saying "wetter is better"? Everyone can use lube anytime they have sex, no matter what kind of sex you're having. It makes both parties more comfortable. It's also great to keep handy because, if you're having vaginal sex and you're going hard, a vagina's natural lubrication cannot keep up with marathon sessions. So lube it up. Refer to our previous thoughts on lubricant for what kind you should add to your collection.

Condoms

So you're about to have sex, it's go time, you're ready, your partner is ready, and you can't find a condom. Insert buzz kill. Keep internal or external condoms handy in a side table, drawer, or brazenly in a bowl next to your bed. Because when the time comes, you want to be ready.

Also, unless you're in a fluid bonded relationship, I would highly recommend using a condom or dental dam every time you engage in sexual activity. The peace of mind you get from reducing your risk of STIs and pregnancy is enough to warrant the minor drawbacks that some say condoms bring. Don't let a thin, thin, thin piece of latex be the thing that stops you from protecting yourself because "It doesn't feel as good." You're getting sex, right? Be happy about that! For those with penises: For an added sensation, add a drop of lube into the tip of the condom before you put it on. Maybe ask your partner to put it on with their mouth. How erotic is that?

Towels

This may sound silly, because you've probably got towels in the bathroom, but again, this is about not having to break the scene to do the naked scavenger hunt. Sex can be messy from sweat and other fluids. A towel can also protect your sheets if you're using oil-based lube, which can make tricky stains that are difficult to remove in the wash. Don't go for that wrinkly old shirt next to your bed! Have a towel nearby and ready. This also is a perfect way to show your tender side, by doing a little aftercare for your partner.

Moist Wipes

Not trying to sound redundant (I know I just mentioned towels), but there is only so much clean-up a dry towel can give. Some bodily fluids, lubes, and other substances can only be cleaned up with the combined wetness and towel-like qualities of a moist wipe. Nothing is worse than having some crusty residue left on your skin. Don't go to bed sticky—no one wants to wake up with an unintentional superhero cape. I'd recommend using a variety specifically made for post-sex clean-up. And remember, throw them away! They do not go into the toilet.

Water

You wouldn't go work out without some form of hydration, right? Sex is a workout too, so treat it like one! During bouts of passion, you're burning tons of calories and losing much of your water through sweat. Help replenish your dehydrated cells by drinking water before, during, and after your sexual activities. This is especially important if you're looking for extended hours of play because if you are dehydrated you will tire more easily. Besides keeping you hydrated, it's great to have water near just to swish around your mouth to rid you of any errant tastes you may have in there.

Toilet Paper

Make sure you have this in the bathroom. You never know when the need may arise for you or your partner. I've been there before—I'm peeing after sex and there is zero toilet paper in my date's bathroom. Like, how are you living like this! (Unless it's a pandemic, #COVID19) Just make sure the bathroom is equipped with paper products for clean-up or otherwise.

Candle

Having a candle burning in the bathroom can save your eyes from hitting that bright vanity light and blowing out your pupils while you use the facilities. All bathrooms should come with dimmer switches, but alas, here we are. The candle can also subtly cover up any odors that may come from your or your partner's bathroom usage. I'm talking about poop here. We have to be adult about these things, and providing a candle is a nice gesture that someone can use if they need. If not, a book of matches will work in a pinch.

It can also be a great touch to have a candle or two burning in the bedroom, to help with the ambiance and to set the mood. Pick a favorite scent and turn off the lights! Just make sure you keep it away from anything flammable. You want to feed the sexual flames, not ones on your curtains.

SEXTING

Sexting is a great way to add spice and fun to dating. This can be used as a mode of foreplay or a creative way to broach the topic of sex. Thinking about sending off some hot messages to your partner, but don't know where to start? Consider these sexting dos and don'ts:

Check that contact: First and foremost, make sure that you're sending your message to the right person. Double check and triple check the name because sending "Mom" instead of "My Love" a seductive message could end in huge embarrassment or unwanted questions.

Text as you would speak: Don't send off a steamy message if it isn't the way you'd talk. If you say, "I'm going to ride you like a pony," but you never speak like that, your partner could be thrown off. Just be yourself.

Leave something to the imagination: Just like you wouldn't want someone to ruin the ending of a good movie, don't say everything in your texts. The idea of sexting is to build anticipation and desire. A sexpot never reveals all of their secrets.

If you're looking for some inspirations, try starting some sexts off with these lines:

If you were here right now . . .
Whatever you do, don't think about me doing [insert naughty activity] to you right now . . .
I can't stop thinking about . . .
Guess where I wish your lips were right now . . .

HOW TO SEND NUDES

I know a lot of people would caution you against sending naked photos on the internet. We've seen celebrity leaks for years, so if they can't keep their photos safe, what are we supposed to do? For me, I already have nude photos on the internet (thanks Playboy!), so it's not going to be that devastating to me if I have photos leaked. Make peace with the fact that your photos are likely going to go beyond the person you sent them to. If that's something you're okay with, you can look at the positives: naked photos are hot! They say a picture is worth a thousand words, and when you're sexting, this can be the catalyst to take your experience to the next level. When taking naked photos, here are some things to keep in mind.[50]

Don't show your face! This is the most important tip for you to know! As we have seen with celebrities, politicians, and athletes, having your face accompanied with your sexy parts can be damaging. Save yourself the stress by taking

---

50 Please be mindful that it is illegal to take, share, or possess nude photos of individuals under eighteen, even if you're under eighteen yourself.

faceless shots. This way you have some level of anonymity. Get close ups of your hot spots instead.

Know your surroundings: Be mindful about what else is in your photo besides you. No one wants to see the toilet or your dirty laundry during your naked selfies. Clean that shit up!

Lighting: What kind of lighting are you shooting in? Direct, overhead lighting is not the most flattering. It can cast harsh shadows and evoke feelings of a medical visit. The best kind of lighting is soft, indirect lighting. You can use this to your advantage by artistically playing with shadows and setting a sultry scene.

Be cheeky: There's no rule that says you have to only send nudes while sexting. If you find yourself more comfortable sending some photos that hint at nudity, do that! Sometimes those photos can be even hotter because they leave some room for imagination and can build anticipation for seeing all of you in the flesh.

DIRTY TALK

Talking dirty, sexy, naughty, nasty, or whatever you want to call it, can be an exciting way to bring your sex play to the next level. Dirty talk can be intimidating for people because it's not something we've been taught to do. But dirty talk is so effective because it's another way to heighten the moment. A few sexy lines whispered to your partner while you're out and about on a date, hinting at things to come, will definitely have them racing to get you home. And a few naughty phrases moaned during the act can really make things hot.

Hearing positive feedback from your partner can also be a great confidence builder, and the wonderful thing about talking dirty is that there is no wrong way to do it.

I love to advise people to just start slowly. You don't have to say anything crazy or have an entire story planned. Just key in on what feels good. Think about your senses and describe how you feel. Also, if profanity or vulgar language isn't something that you commonly use, don't feel pressured to use it. It might throw your partner off if you're suddenly asking "Master" to "fuck his little cum dumpster."

If you're starting from nothing, dip your toes into the dirty talk pool with some simple moans and groans. Give a sigh or have a catch in your breath. Starting to become vocal in the act will make you more comfortable when it comes time to say it with words.

If you're feeling shy or not sure what to say, just stick to basic phrases. Keep it simple and sexy. Here are some ideas:

You're so sexy.
I love it when you _____ my _____.
Lick me here.
That feels so good.
Touch my [favorite spot].
I'm going to _____ your_____.

These simple phrases and more sound super erotic when said into your partner's ear. Just give them a verbal play by play of what's happening. Tell your partner what you're about to do to them. That will also help keep you present, and keep your mind on task. And everyone loves compliments, especially in the bedroom!

If you're looking to up the ante, try out these lines:

> *Let's see how many times I can make you come.*
> *You're so wet.*
> *You taste delicious.*
> *I love the feeling of you in my mouth.*
> *I'm coming.*
> *Come on my face.*
> *You can put it anywhere.*

As your confidence builds, you can work in more naughty phrases and words into your repertoire. If you and your partner are both comfortable with it, try some vulgarity! Get nasty with it. Also realize that what goes on in the bedroom doesn't necessarily translate into real life. For example, your date might like it when you call them a whore while in the act, but they may not like being called a whore in public. Talking dirty is just for fun and should never be used maliciously against your partner.

You have to be able to laugh off any mistakes you make during dirty talk. They're bound to happen. Sometimes you have a great line in your head, but as it's coming out, it gets jumbled and makes zero sense. Like the one time I told a guy his freckles were cute, just like my mom's. We made awkward eye contact and then laughed.

ORAL SEX

Oral sex is a fun way to connect with a new partner. It can be used as foreplay, or you can make it the main event. Here are some things to keep in mind when exploring oral play.

Be Enthusiastic

Do you really want to be doing this? Your partner can pick up on the energy that you're giving off. Go into this activity with gusto or tell them that you're not feeling up to it right now.

Positions

This is so key! You absolutely do not have to be on your hands and knees, bent over, to perform oral sex. That position can be uncomfortable, especially if on your hands and knees for a prolonged amount of time. You know when your arm starts to shake from holding yourself up? That's what I'm talking about. Move your partner into a position that is comfortable for both of you. I like to recommend that your partner be on an elevated surface where you can comfortably fit between their legs when you're upright on your knees on the floor, with them at a comfortable height so that your face is positioned right at their genitals. Add a pillow or soft cushion below your knees. In this position, your neck is supported and you have two free hands to use on your partner.

One other position for oral sex on a vulva that I'd like to point out is the Kivin method. This is also called sideways oral sex. The partner giving the oral sex will be on either side of the receiver (try out both sides, as people usually have a more sensitive side of their clitoris). The giving partner should lie on their side perpendicular to the receiving partner. They can then open the labia and begin to lick back and forth over the hood of the clitoris. With a free hand, the giver can apply pressure to the perineum (the taint). As the receiving partner becomes more aroused, the giver should be able to feel some preorgasmic contractions. Should be quite pleasurable!

Use Your Hands

And speaking of hands, use them! Just because this is oral sex it doesn't mean that you can't tag in a hand to help. Adding variety in stimulation and pressure with your hands and mouth makes for a more dynamic oral experience. This can also be helpful if you have a partner who has a particularly large penis or is into prostate stimulation.

Use a Toy

Just like adding hands, adding a toy can up level your oral sex game. A toy is a great tool to use during oral because it won't get tired out like a human body part. A bullet vibrator is my go-to for this. Toys can also be used to stimulate other hotspots (like nipples and perineum) while you're giving oral sex. This is also an opportunity to explore anal play during oral sex (flared base toy only!).

Be Spontaneous

Knowing that you have sex on Tuesday, Thursday, and the weekend can be good for planning purposes, but spice things up with some surprise oral sometimes. Try to do it in an unexpected location, like when your partner is brushing their teeth (obviously with consent). The novelty of the new experience will have your partner excited and keep them on their toes.

Show Your Partner What to Do

Getting to know new bodies can be tricky, so if you're the recipient of oral sex, give your partner some help. Show your partner the ways in which you like to be touched. I'm not suggesting a lecture format with a PowerPoint slide, but rather, an opportunity for you to explore together.

As for how to do this: If the conversation feels natural, consider bringing it up as you're getting to know them. Ask open-ended questions like, "Tell me some of the ways you like to be turned on." Or you can literally come out and say, "If you fist your hand in my hair, tilt my head back, and kiss up my neck, chances are I will spontaneously combust."

If you think that actions are stronger than words, then consider letting your partner watch you touch yourself during play, which will help show them what turns you on. Alternatively, you can guide their head with your hands.

Ask for Feedback

It's always a good idea to check in with your partner during oral sex, particularly if you are the one giving. Ask them for feedback. "Do you like this touch? Where do you want me to touch you? Would you like it if I . . . ?" The more you're able to get specific details on what drives your partner wild, the better able you will be to please them.

Giving Oral Sex

Psych yourself up! Especially if you're nervous. Chances are that your partner is going to like whatever you're about to do to them. They probably have some nervous anticipation too. Remind yourself that this isn't a race. There's no time limit on how long a person "should" take to reach orgasm. Also, remember the fact that orgasm isn't required to have an enjoyable sexual encounter. Learning a new partner's body takes time, and there will be a learning curve. You aren't going to do everything just as they like it the first time. Where would the fun in that be? They're just happy to have you between their legs! A great sexual experience should be a giving and receiving of sexual pleasure between two people who honor each other.

Start off slowly and ease and tease your way into the stimulation. Feel free to take breaks, ask for feedback, and take your time.

Receiving Oral Sex

Give them a round of applause! But for real, you can do whatever you want while receiving oral sex. You can use this time to play with your partner's head or hair, whether that is controlling the position of their head or giving them a scalp massage. You can also rub up on your own exposed skin, assuming you are topless. Pinching your nipples can be an erotic sensation when coupled with oral play. You can also do your own take on the savasana pose in yoga, with your palms turned up and your head back, and just surrender to the sensation.

Sometimes auditory cues like moans or words of encouragement can help let your partner know that they're on the right track. Don't be over the top though—be authentic in your sounds.

WORRIED ABOUT TASTE

Sometimes people (especially those with vaginas) are hesitant to engage in oral sex due to worries about how they will taste. The taste of your vagina can vary throughout your cycle and can be influenced by what you've been eating and drinking. If the taste seems overly strong or it has a strong foul odor, you may consider seeking out medical attention, as you may have a bacterial condition or an STI. The vagina is self-cleaning, so it is important to stay properly hydrated in order for that to take place. There is also a delicate balance of bacteria inside of your vagina, and the slightest shift in the environment can send things askew.

I recommend that you taste yourself if you have concerns about whether your natural flavor is unpalatable. Adding more things to your diet like water, fruits, and vegetables has anecdotally been shown to improve vaginal taste. Otherwise, if your partner cannot get behind going down on you, or you feel too self-conscious to let them, try oral sex fresh from a shower and/or use a dental dam.

When cleansing your vulva, pure water is great! There are also pH-balanced washes that are specifically made for your genital region. Do not use regular soap. This can disrupt your ecosystem, leading to even more odors and potential infection. Even if you're using the correct pH-balanced soap, this is for external washing only. Nothing should be going inside of your vagina. This is why we (the sex educators) caution against using douches. Douches disrupt your vagina's balance of bacteria, and then the bad bacteria come back with a vengeance.

If you're a penis owner, mild, gentle soap is recommended for your parts as well. Too much washing or use of harsh soaps can lead to skin irritations. If there's a persistent odor that is not your normal scent, there's a chance you may have some kind of infection. Best to seek out medical attention, not to add more flowery-smelling soaps.

EJACULATE IN THE EYE

Two fast fun facts about ejaculate in the eyeball: One, it can remove lash extensions! My lash lady told me that. Also, if you use artificial tanner, it can leave you with some pretty unique splash patterns (aka eat away your fake tan). I'm not a self-tanner, but I am a lash extension user, so no facials here.

As far as how long the pain will last when you get ejaculate in the eye, it is really up to your body's reaction. First and foremost, try to flush out your eye with water as soon as possible. It may feel like there is some serious damage to your eye, but it just usually ends up being irritated for a while. The longer the ejaculate is in the eye, the longer/stronger the symptoms can be. The symptoms should clear up on their own, so a doctor's visit usually isn't necessary. Of course, if you're experiencing long-lasting symptoms or trouble with your vision, seek out a medical professional.

PENIS WON'T STAY HARD

This is a common concern when dealing with erections. Don't worry if your erection comes and goes, or if your partner's erection comes and goes. This is a bodily function, and sometimes bodies have minds of their own. Do not equate a partner's erection with arousal, like some kind of cock-o-meter, meaning that if they're losing an erection or going soft that they're losing interest in you. Men will tell you that any kind of stimulation on their penis, hard or soft, feels good. You can still have a fun and satisfying sexual encounter without an erection.

Try not to make a big deal of it. Penises do not respond to nervous pressure well. Nerves can just exacerbate the situation. If your partner loses the erection, just continue with what you were doing or move on to a different activity. Chances are that the erection will return—but even if it doesn't, that's perfectly okay. Check in with your partner and ask if they'd prefer a different touch, or if what you're currently doing to them feels nice. They are the masters of their penis, and they will be able to point you in the right direction.

And if you happen to be the penis owner, know that it's okay! Erections come and go, and there is nothing you can do about it. Don't feel like you have to apologize for how your body performs. Erections, or the loss of them, are not indicative of how aroused or turned on you are from your partner.

FINGERING

While penetration can be a pleasurable sensation, around 75% of women require clitoral stimulation to reach orgasm, so don't be dismayed if you or your partner aren't climaxing from penetration alone. Here are some tips for giving manual stimulation.

If you're going to engage in some manual play, consider starting off with some general external touching of the vulva to warm things up, and then lead off penetration with one finger first. If you think they want another, ask first! Unless you're a mind reader, the only way to be sure that another finger would be welcome is to ask your partner. Once you start to learn your partner's body and their likes and dislikes, you will get a better sense of whether or not an additional finger is welcome.

The G-spot (or rather, G-area), can be found on the anterior wall of the vagina. So if your partner is lying on their back, you can locate this area by inserting a lubricated finger in with your palm up. The tissue should feel engorged when aroused and different from the surrounding tissue. You can use a "come hither" motion with your finger, running along the inside of the vagina, or some light percussive tapping with the pad of your finger.

With lubricated fingers you can approach the clitoris gently. Ask your partner what kind of touch, stroke, intensity, and positioning they enjoy. Some touches might include rubbing around the clitoral head, slipping your fingers between the labia, or spreading the labia apart with one hand and using the other to have direct access to the vagina.

Even though the vagina is self-lubricating, it's always great to have lubrication on hand. Sometimes your partner may not lubricate enough for painless penetration, and that is completely normal. It isn't an indication that they are less into you or aren't as turned on. Sometimes bodies need extra help.

One of the biggest tips I can suggest for stepping up your fingering game is to slow it down. So often, activities like fingering are an afterthought or just a short prelude to the main event of PV sex. Take your time and make this its own activity to be enjoyed. If given enough time and the right stimulation, you can help your partner to orgasm many times over and keep them glowing for days.

PENETRATIVE SEX POSITIONS

Penetrative sex is arguably one of the closest ways you can connect with someone. And penetrative sex can include many activities, such as PV (penis in vagina) sex, use of a strap-on, and anal play. Whether this is your first time or you're a veteran, having sex with someone new is always an exciting experience. You're discovering how they like to be pleasured and how the two of you work together. Sometimes one position doesn't work out for us, and that can be discouraging. Luckily, there are an almost infinite number of sex positions for all types of bodies and abilities. Here are some that you can try with your partner.

Missionary

This classic sex position is where the penetrator is on top and the partners are face-to-face. This is great for maximum body contact and for looking into each other's eyes. The receptive partner has the ability to use their hands to stimulate themselves, use a toy, or run them along their partner's body. By controlling the opening of their legs, they can also limit how much penetration is available to the penetrating partner.

Spooning

This sex position is done while lying in the spooning position (both partners on their sides). The penetrating partner enters from behind. This position is great if either of you have back pain, as it is very low impact. The penetration is not as deep as in other positions, but the freedom both partners have to touch and caress each other makes this a hot configuration. This position can be modified by the receiver bending their knees to allow deeper access. The penetrating partner can spread the receivers butt cheeks or legs to facilitate this.

Coital Alignment Technique: CAT

This position is set up the same way missionary is except that the penetrator is higher on the body of the receiver. This position is designed to have maximum clitoral stimulation. The penetrator should comfortably rest their weight on the receiver, and everyone should relax their muscles. Their pelvises should be aligned. Penetration will now slide against the clitoris.

Rear Entry

Sometimes called doggy-style, this position is great if you want to have a little more freedom to move. In this position, the penetrator has entered the receiver from behind. Both people are on their knees. Both partners have the freedom to stimulate each other in a variety of ways. The penetrator can pull the receiver's hair (gently!), put a finger in the butt, or even reach around to play with their nipples. The receiver can self-stimulate. This position can be modified for a variety of body types and abilities. You can modify this position to work on a couch, the stairs, or even a table. The penetrator can be standing as well. Lots of opportunities for this position.

Yab Yum

This is a classic Tantra pose that is great for turning up the intimacy and connection. The penetrator will sit in a crossed legged position on the bed. The receiver will climb on top of the legs of the penetrator and wrap their legs around the torso of the penetrator. They can adjust themselves as needed. This position encourages closeness. Partners can look into each other's eyes, hug, kiss, or even use a toy between their bodies.

Cowgirl

This position refers to when the receiver is on top of the penetrator. This is often cited as a favorite position for women because they're able to stimulate their clitoris by rubbing against their partner's pelvis. Also, riding your partner can be empowering—the person below gets an amazing show and can stimulate you while you're doing so.

Have the penetrator lay down on their back on the bed. The receiver mounts their partner. They can assume a kneeling position or stay on their feet in a deep squat, whatever they're in the mood for.

Journal prompt: What are some positions that you have tried? Which did you like best, and why? What are some positions that you want to try? What about those positions sounds appealing?

PAINFUL SEX

As we've discussed, many people suffer in silence over painful sex. I think this issue stems from a lack of comprehensive sex education. Many people inadvertently supplement their sex education by taking in media like TV and porn, and they think what they see on screen is like real life. No one is reaching for lube when the sex scene starts! And most definitely, no one is saying the sex hurts unless it's for comedic effect.

One common cause of pain during sex is a lack of sufficient lubricant. Lubricant is a normal, healthy component of someone's sex life. Depending on the sex you're having, certain parts do not produce their own natural lubricant. And even the vagina has a finite amount of lubricant that it can produce during one session. Sometimes people view the use of additional lube as a reflection of their inability to turn on their partner. But I'll say it again: There is no correlation between arousal and lubrication level. Yes, those two things often happen together, but it's not a rule. Sometimes things like medication, age, or environmental factors can impact someone's natural lubrication. They may still be very turned on, but just not lubricating. It's totally normal.

Lubricant is a part of a healthy sex life. I love a water-based lubricant like Doc Johnson's water-based mood lubricant. It is condom and toy friendly, plus very easy to clean up! If you're looking to engage in anal play, you most definitely need lubricant because the anus does not naturally lubricate.

Consider using a silicone-based lubricant for longevity. It is more viscous than water-based lube and is still condom friendly.

But there are also other reasons why sex may be painful. I don't think people talk about painful sex because there is an aura of shame around it. Those who are affected by it often internalize those feelings rather than take the chance of hurting their partner's feelings. And this can feel especially tricky when dating someone new.

Painful sex can be caused by a variety of factors, including a lack of lubrication, the wrong size/fit of an external condom, vaginismus, phimosis, UTIs, Bartholin's glands cysts, vestibulitis or vulvodynia, balanitis, STIs, or other body injuries.

Painful sex can happen to anyone! People of every gender can experience pain during sex for many different reasons, and it's not something to be ashamed of. No partner is a mind reader, so it's important to communicate what's going on with you to a partner. There are many treatment options like physical therapy, medications, and products people can use to help mitigate pain during sex if it is beyond a problem with the position or a lack of lubrication. Be open to trying many ways to find what works best for you.

SEX INJURIES

These things can happen. There is even a whole TV show dedicated to this called, *Sex Sent Me to the ER*. Here are some common things to be on the lookout for:

Rug Burn

Rug burn can happen when there is vigorous friction of your skin against a fabric. Think carpet or rough upholstery. You may not feel it in the moment, but after sex these injuries can present themselves. As long as they are just superficial, you are okay to treat them with simple first aid.

Vaginal Bleeding

Vaginal lacerations can happen from rough sex and/or lack of lubrication. This can occur because of vaginal penetration by fingers, a penis, or a toy. The tissues of the vagina normally lubricate, but sometimes it isn't enough for penetration to be pain free. Small tears will heal on their own, but if a tear continues to bleed, it's time to seek medical attention.

Broken Penis

While there are no bones in a penis, you can still get what's referred to as a "penis fracture" from rough play. Think next level terrible bruise! It happens when the tunica that surrounds the spongy, blood-filled corpora cavernosa tissue literally tears and releases blood, often due to a blunt force. This is something that you have to seek medical attention to treat. Best to ice it and head to the ER.

Head Trauma

Shower sex always seems like a good idea until someone slips. Even if you aren't having penetrative sex, the chances of you slipping and hitting your head or breaking a bone is still there. If you have any doubts about the severity of your injury, it's best to seek medical attention.

Infections

Bacterial infections are very common and with treatment can be cured relatively quickly. These can happen when there is an imbalance of the good and bad bacteria in your vagina. Best practices are to have clean hands and toys before you begin your play, and to urinate after sex to flush out any recently introduced bacteria.

Something Got Lost

Getting items stuck or lost is a pretty common occurrence. If something is lost in the vagina, it won't be lost forever. As the vagina is closed off from the rest of the body via the cervix, it just takes some maneuvering to remove any objects (condoms, tampons, toys). You may need assistance from your partner. The rectum is a different issue. If you are playing with a toy or object in the rectum, it MUST be attached to a body or have a flared base. Without a base, without a trace. If you lose something in your rectum, you have to seek medical attention to have it removed (See the sex toys section in Chapter 3 for a list of items people have lost in their butts.)

CHAPTER 11:
WORST CASE SCENARIO
SURVIVAL GUIDE

ook, sometimes dating can be a hot mess. You can plan and plan, but sometimes the universe has something else in store for you. You should be prepared for anything. There are plenty of books with advice on what to do when a date goes wrong, like, "If you and your partner cannot pay your bill, prepare to wash the dishes." I'm over here telling you the stuff that's not in those books, like how to deal with that Mentos and diet cola intestinal explosion that's about to ruin your date, and quite possibly, your pants.

YOU HAVE GAS ON A DATE

This tip has honestly saved me so many times on a date or while at my date's house. This is assuming that you two aren't yet at the level of being cool with letting farts fly. If you have gas, excuse yourself to go to the bathroom. Get down on all fours and assume the Downward Dog yoga position. This is where you have both your feet and hands on the ground with your ass in the air. We're trying to help the gas escape and exit up and out. If you find yourself in a public bathroom, lay some paper towel down, lest you return to the table covered in bathroom grime. You should be able to feel the gas moving. Sway back and forth to expedite the departure. When you return, casually order some peppermint tea to calm down your stomach. Ginger candy can also help with this.

YOU FORGOT TO SHAVE

We all learned what a rushed shave job can end up like. Floss anyone? Shaving is totally optional (and that goes for shaving any part of your body). You have the right to present your body however you like, and you do not need to change yourself to satisfy a date or partner. But if you do feel more comfortable shaved, you have a few options here. You can quickly do a rush shave job and hope that you did a good enough rinse job and call it good. You can say fuck it, and show up as is (honestly, they don't care!). Or you can ask your partner to shave you!

BAD KISSER

It's wet, it's wide open, and I don't think I can take another minute of it. If this is your experience, gently grab your partner's head and pull it away from yours. Ask them if you can show them how you like to be kissed. The answer should be an enthusiastic yes. Slow it down and try again. Kiss them the way you like to be kissed, and then let them try. Give them praise when they're doing a good job. And remember: It's not necessarily a failing on their part. You never know, their previous partner could have loved it like this.

SHIT! I FORGOT THEIR NAME!

If for whatever reason you forgot the name of the person you had sex with, there are a few options to save yourself with. Go to the bathroom and see if you can find any prescription bottles with their name on it. Just don't get caught because then you look like a weirdo searching for drugs. Check their coffee table for mail or magazine subscriptions. And if those lead you nowhere, "babe" is a good catchall.

PENIS IS TOO BIG

I like a challenge as much as the next person, but sometimes you come across a penis of the XL variety. First of all, don't panic. Let's remember that vaginas are super dynamic and can open to the size of a baby. This is a time to not skimp on the foreplay. The more relaxed and aroused you are, the more your vagina will be able to tent. Take it slowly. Use a finger or two to open you up and only when you're ready dive in for penetration.

You may also want to add more lubricant—whatever you can do to ease entry. Stick to positions that limit the amount of penetration like spooning, cowgirl or reverse cowgirl, yab yum, or stacked spoons (where you lay on your stomach with your legs together and your partner slides in-between your thighs to enter you). Don't write off a guy just because he has a large piece. You can work with whatever they've got.

YOU'RE ON YOUR PERIOD

Well first of all, mention that you're on your period. If that's something that you're both cool with, go ahead! Lay a towel down to take care of any fluid leakage, and remember that just because you're on your period doesn't mean that you can't get pregnant.

If you're not both interested in having vaginal sex, you can engage in other activities like sensual massage or anal sex.

QUESTIONS FROM THE AUDIENCE

Here is a sampling of questions I have received from my audience over the years.

How Do I Shave My Vagina?

Well technically we are shaving our vulva, but I know what you meant. Save your time (and razor) by giving yourself a trim with scissors first if your hair is quite long. When you start using a razor for a closer shave, make sure you have a shaving cream or conditioner to use as a buffer between your razor and skin. Shave with the growth of your hair (in the same direction it grows). If you go against the grain, you run the risk of having ingrown hairs. Those itch, and it's probably not the best look to be itching your crotch before your next sexual encounter. Shaving is totally optional. You can absolutely let your hair, anywhere, grow as long as you like.

Is Anal Safe? What Can I Do to Prepare for Anal?

Anal sex is a totally safe sex practice when done correctly. To prepare for anal, I suggest you take a shower and wash your butt. Just to get rid of any loose hairs, residue, or errant toilet paper (this has happened before, don't judge me). Some people like to do an internal cleaning with an enema. This is where you flush out the lower portion of your rectum (see below for tips). Once you're clean and ready, make sure you have plenty of lubricant on hand, and that you've discussed safer sex practices. Take things slowly, and you can even try working your way up to penetration with a penis by using smaller toys intended for anal play.

How to Do an Enema

Fleet enemas are readily available at any supermarket or drugstore. Make sure you are purchasing a simple saline one and NOT one that is oil based or contains a laxative.

When you get home, first make sure you have a bowel movement before using the enema. Then I want you to unscrew the bottle and dump the contents down the drain. Stay with me here. Even though you may have purchased a plain saline enema, it can still contain some laxative agents. Refill your bottle with warm well-filtered or distilled water. Don't just use tap water. We want to avoid cold water because it can make you cramp, and hot water can burn your insides. We want the goldilocks porridge temperature.

Once you've refilled your bottle, you can either lie on your side with your knees curled up or you can get on all fours to insert the liquid into your anus. Wait five minutes and release the liquid into the toilet. You can repeat the process a few times until the water is clear. If you use too much liquid (don't use more than one bottle, or the amount recommended by the product you purchased) or wait too long (you'll know this if not enough liquid comes out, based on the amount that went in), you could inadvertently be giving yourself a deep enema, which means you'd have to put all butt play on hold. With a deep enema, you're going to have some leakage.

But let's say that you did everything correctly and you're ready to go—awesome! Wait about a half hour for the remaining water in your rectum to be absorbed, and then go have fun!

How Can I Get Out of My Head During Sex? I Can't Stop Thinking about My Insecurities

Getting out of your head during sex can be a challenge if you're struggling with some insecurities, but there are things you can do to help. First of all, ask yourself if there is anything you can change to make you more comfortable in the moment. Maybe that's only doing certain positions, where you feel at your best. Maybe that means only having candlelight. It really depends on what insecurities you've got going on.

If there isn't anything immediate to be done about your insecurities, you can focus in on the sensations your body is feeling. Take a deep breath. Take another. What do you feel? What can you hear? What can you taste? What can you smell? What can you see? Lean in to those sensations and try to get lost in them. Find a sense of presence (being in the moment) within those senses, and your insecurities should start to become background noise.

Sure you might not like the way your stomach hangs when you are on top, but oh my god your partner's mouth on your nipple while their hard cock is inside you can eclipse that worry. Also, trust that your partner finds you attractive and wants to be with you—otherwise, they would not be there with you.

My Vagina Is Sore for Days After Penetrative Sex. How Do I Avoid This?

Vaginal soreness can come from a variety of causes. Maybe you had sex with a large penis (see above). If this is happening on the regular, your body will adjust to your partner's size and eventually it shouldn't be an issue. Maybe you had some rough sex. This can totally make you sore, as more aggressive, deeper penetration can light up places in your body that don't normally see any action. Try to remember if you engaged in anything specifically that might have caused this. Either way, try to slow down and spend more time on foreplay.

How Do You Use Lube?

This might seem like an obvious question, but there are a variety of ways that you can use lube. If you're using lube for solo play, you can apply the lube to your fingers or directly onto the desired location. Depending on the kind of lube you're using, it may be easy or difficult to keep it in the place that you want it. If using a toy, apply the lubricant directly to the toy. You don't want to get snagged on a dry part of the toy. If you're going to engage in penetrative sex with a partner, lube both of you up. If you're struggling to get the lube to go where you want, you can purchase a lube shooter. It's a syringe that you can fill, insert into an orifice, and depress the plunger to have lube right where you need it. What a time to be alive.

How Can I Last Longer in Bed?

To last longer in bed, you can always try edging (see Chapter 5) to extend your play. You can also switch positions frequently. Think beyond the bounds of penetrative sex, and how long you might last if you start including other things like oral sex and massage. And even if you do happen to come before you want to, that doesn't mean that the play has to stop. You can continue to play with your partner. Depending on your refractory period (the time it takes for you to become aroused again), you may be able to have another sexual release if you continue.

Does the Number of Partners I've Had Matter?

The question to be asking is, "Does the number of partners matter to me?" If it does, ask yourself why? I'm all about eliminating sexual shame, and that comes with ending judgment on someone's sexual past. If it's a matter of safety, getting tested and asking your partner to do the same is an easy way to allay any fears or concerns you may have. Otherwise, a number is just a number in my opinion.

What if I Look Ugly Down There?

First of all, ugly according to whom? Vulvas are as varied as snowflakes. They come in many different shapes, colors, and textures. Penises are just as varied. If you think you're ugly because your body varies from mainstream porn, you're wrong to believe that. We've been conditioned to recognize one type of vulva as "hot" because that's what we commonly see, if we see any vulvas at all. Hairless, small labia, and pink. When in reality, vulvas can have gradients of colors, can have lips that hang, can be asymmetrical, and can certainly be hairy. There are some great resources like *Vulva 101* by Hylton Coxwell or *Petals* by Nick Karras that can help you see the variation on vulvas. They're all beautiful. If you're a penis owner, check out the book *Manhood: The Bare Reality*, which features photos of one hundred penises and stories from their owners on their journey to body acceptance.

What Do I Do if Someone I Like Is Still Caught Up on Their Ex?

If someone you like is still caught up on their ex, the best thing you can do is give them space to figure things out with their ex. If you jump into a relationship with them right now, and there are still unresolved issues with their ex, you've got a relationship starting on rocky ground. People need time to heal, recover, and regroup after a breakup. There is nothing wrong with putting things on pause while some time passes. If they are pressuring you into a relationship, talk to them and explain where your head's at with all of this. Use I statements, and hold firm. If things are resolved and you still have mutual interest, go for it!

What Do I Say to Family Members Who Make Comments about My Size?

This comment is quite common, especially around the holidays. It's usually followed or preceded by comments about when you're going to be in a relationship *insert eyeroll*. You can deal with this in a variety of ways. You can have a preemptive conversation with your family and ask that there be no talk about body size or diet. You can say you're grateful for their concern, but then tell them why what they're saying is hurtful. You can throw some science at them (for instance, you need fat to survive, for warmth, and for organ protection). You can also say that you're trying to heal your relationship with food, and comments like that are detrimental to your progress. And ultimately, you don't have to go to whatever function it is where you know a family member there will talk about your body.

CONCLUSION

Here we are friends. Thank you for sticking with me through this journey. I hope you can stand tall in your truth and pursue your dreams. I want you to cultivate your hobbies, be brave, try new things, feel good about yourself, and most importantly be your own best lover. No one knows what the future holds for us, but I hope that you feel a little more secure in the fact that you're ready to face whatever this world throws at you.

Even if you don't feel ready to jump into everything I've covered here, I want you to know that right now, right this very second, as you read these words, you are enough. You deserve to have happiness and to have your desires met. There is really no ending when it comes to cultivating a life of contentment and sexual fulfillment. There is just the journey. Trust the reroute when something doesn't go your way, and just keep going. Life is a rollercoaster filled with twists and turns, scary drops, and soaring highs. Remind yourself daily to enjoy the ride because life is never linear, and neither is a good ride. 😉

ACKNOWLEDGMENT

would like to express my deepest appreciation to Hannah Bennett. My success in bringing this book to life would not have been possible without her nurturing support and kind words to this fledgling author. I'm also extremely grateful for her keen editing eye that was instrumental in making this book flow effortlessly.

I cannot begin to express my thanks to Jessica O'Reilly. Thank you for in connecting me with the wonderful people at Cleis, and for always being a pillar of support and encouragement throughout my career. I am so honored to call you a friend.

I would also like to extend my sincere thanks to the rest of the team at Cleis for their hard work in making this book a reality.

The reality is that writing a book is difficult and without the support of my community of friends and loved ones, this book may very well still be in the rough outline state that it began with. Thank you Stephanie, Jennie, Diane, Mary Lynne, Kelsey, Sarah, Chris, Justine, Janene, Hyuibin, Dave,

Baby Joe, Brad, Sailesh, and Joyce for the emotional, spiritual, and moral support. Whether it was keeping me to task, reminding me of laughable stories from my colorful past, or hyping me up when I was down and convinced that no one would want to read this book, I am indebted to you all. I am strong because you stand beside me and build me up with love. I'd also like to extend my gratitude to Mom. Thank you for teaching me to read at a young age and never saying no when it came to book purchases.

A special thank you to those teachers and professors who helped me fall in love with science and sex even more than I already did. Many thanks to my colleagues as well. And I would be remiss if I didn't mention the amazing strangers who I don't know by name that have attended my events over the years. Thank you college students, retreat attendees, workshop participants, and readers afar. You're the reason I do what I do.

And Kronos, I love you.